ELECTRO-ACUPUNCTURE FOR DENTISTRY

BY JOHN K. CHAR, D.D.S.

EAV SPECIAL

DR. JOHN K. CHAR • HOLISTIC DENTISTRY • 1980

The author is deeply grateful to Dr. Reinhold Voll, M.D.
for his contribution and his understanding in using his great works for this chapter.
Without his cooperation, this chapter would not have been possible.

Special gratitude should also be given to Dr. Willem Khoe, M.D.
who has helped to spread Voll's work in
holistic dentistry and medicine in America today.

Table of Contents*

HOLISTIC DENTISTRY

VOLUME ONE

EAV SPECIAL

VOLUME TWO

* Table Of Contents For Page Numbers Located At The Inside Bottom Corner Of Each Page

Table of Contents

EAV SPECIAL • Electro-Acupuncture for Dentistry

INTRODUCTION TO ELECTRO-ACUPUNCTURE BY VOLL

DIAGNOSTIC EVALUATION OF THE MANAGEMENT CRITERIA

THE DERMATRON

OPERATING INSTRUCTIONS FOR THE EAV

PATIENT MANAGEMENT IN EAV

HAND ELECTRO-ACUPUNCTURE POINTS ACCORDING TO VOLL

FOOT ELECTRO-ACUPUNCTURE POINTS ACCORDING TO VOLL

BODY ELECTRO-ACUPUNCTURE POINTS ACCORDING TO VOLL

YIN AND YANG PRINCIPLE OF OPPOSITES

ENERGETIC REACTIONS BETWEEN THE ODONTONS AND THE ORGANS AND TISSUE SYSTEMS

DENTAL THERAPY

BIBLIOGRAPHY

INTRODUCTION TO ELECTRO-ACUPUNCTURE BY VOLL

Voll and his Work

Dr. Voll was born in Berlin on February 17, 1909, the son of an architect. The young Voll soon developed an interest in technology and as a radio amateur during his high school years laid the foundations for his later research in electro-acupuncture. After graduating from high school, he followed in his father's footsteps and took up studies in architecture at the Technical University of Stuttgart, only to find that medicine was his real vocation. His interest during his medical studies at the Universities of Tuebingen and Hamburg soon focused on anatomy. It is only with a sound basis in human anatomy that modern acupuncture can be practiced effectively.

During his medical career, Dr. Voll engaged in preventive medicine both in industry and child welfare, and finally becoming a medical practitioner in southern Germany in 1943. As early as 1953 he began practicing electro-acupuncture and since 1959 has devoted his entire medical activity to this newly developed science.

In 1956 he founded and actually promoted the Association for Electro-acupuncture which became an international organization in 1961 with Dr. Voll as the president until 1972, when he became honorary president.

The association, with members in more than 17 countries, offers training courses for medical doctors and dentists and has held more than 120 such courses in electro-acupuncture diagnostics and therapy, in addition to workshops and scientific sessions mainly in Germany.

Ever since 1961, electro-acupuncture has been gaining more and more dedicated followers, proving that Dr. Voll's far-reaching concepts opened the gates for new significant approaches in medical diagnostics and therapy.

I had an opportunity to visit Dr. Voll's office in Plochigen, Germany. After a week's observation of Voll's method of treatment on patients from all sectors of the world, I concluded that his method of treatment encompassed a holistic approach of preventive and comprehensive diagnosis and treatment not found in orthodox medicine today. Within 15 minutes of the visit, the patient is tested on the Dermatron at over 20 acupuncture meridians on the hands and feet. By the use of low frequency alternating electric current, Dr. Voll was able to tonify irritated acupuncture foci points to improve the body's energy in degenerative organs or sedate points of inflammation to their normal physiological values. By matching homeopathic remedies from plants, minerals, animal and nosodes (energy from diseased tissues), he was able to induce similar potencies into the body. In effect, this produced a stimuli within the body to act on the cause and initiate the body's defensive mechanism to react and withdraw its own disease from within. Each organ and dysfunction was treated with homeopathic remedies. Within a three week period, most of the causative problems were under control and many irritated foci of infections were back to a normal physiological balance. Of great importance is the dental foci of infections which can be the cause of 90% of organ tissue, joint and vertebrae dysfunction. This will be explained in more detail in this chapter. EAV has introduced new concepts in dentistry and expanded the role of preventive health and nutrition especially in the diagnosis and treatment for dental stress.

Dr. Willem Khoe, a noted surgeon for twenty years from Sun Valley, California, is America's leading authority on holistic medicine. His use of electro-acupuncture by Voll, classical acupuncture, sonopuncture, aquapuncture, biomagnetics, basic and Oriental herbology, nutrition, exercises and homeopathic remedies are all combined to treat the whole person rather than only symptoms. His continual research with the Acupuncture Research Institute and his teaching principles have been instrumental in fostering the use of total preventive health concepts among his colleagues and those in the dental profession in the United States.

Public sentiment in favor of the natural sciences are influencing today's total health picture. This has created alterations to allopathic standards as to the mode of treatment. Although there is still strong opposition to this discipline from certain entrenched circles of medicine and dentistry; the results of Voll and Khoe's accomplishments will set standards for future generations. These two men have the vision to use the age-old concepts of acupuncture, biomagnetics, herbs, etc., and to modify them with highly technical and scientific methodology in order to diagnose, treat and ultimately cure diseases and dysfunctions of the human body. This, in effect is the difference between crisis medicine and preventive health practice. Their work measures the exact natural remedy which stimulates the body's defensive mechanism to ward off the disease rather than act as a suppressor like so many of the chemical drugs used today. In other words, they have enabled the body to heal itself rather than let the drug do the work. Their method treats and prevents disease in its early stage halting its progress on to a degenerative stage rather than overwhelming, depressing and irritating the vital organs.

The following chapter gives a basic explanation of the Dermatron and its application to other disciplines. Don't assume that this instrument will cure all. However, this machine when used as a tool to make an accurate diagnosis, helps the doctor care for that individual's immediate needs long enough for the body to actively heal and repair itself. It will take intensive training, patience, dedication and perseverance to thoroughly understand and use this instrument to accomplish the above goals. It is recommended that those interested in expanding their knowledge in electro-acupuncture by Voll, take Voll and Khoe's instructive courses.

For further information on Voll's work, write to:

The American Journal of Acupuncture • 1400 Lost Acre Drive • Felton, California 95018

Voll's five volumes in English can be ordered at the International Scholarly Book Services, Inc., P.O. Box 555, Forest Grove, Oregon 97116.

For more information on Khoe's work, write to:

Willem H. Khoe, M.D. • 9375 San Fernando Road • Sun Valley, California 91352 • Phone: (213) 768-3000

Introduction

Today, dentistry is recognized as a highly specialized field of medicine since dental pathology has been shown to have a definite correlation to organs, glands, joints, bones and vertebrae. In order to treat the local manifestation of the disease in the mouth, it is important to consider treating the general physical state of the patient. Voll's *Interrelations of Odontons and Tonsils to Organs, Fields of Disturbance and Tissue Systems* clearly shows the importance of the dentist's role in health prevention.

Voll used a modification of classical homeopathy. He surmised that every substance, animate or inanimate, has an electromagnetic field. Taking the ancient art of traditional Chinese acupuncture, he developed his technique with an instrument called the Dermatron. This device enabled the doctor to measure the acupuncture points where a small energetic barrage is formed where an energetic potential of the respective organ can be measured or influenced. These loci possess electric potential differing from the surrounding surface of the skin.

In addition to the above, energy produced in one organ is not stored but rather passed on to the entire body. The energy generated in the body, by some sort of circulation, passes through the whole body in a diurnal rhythm through certain pathways, called the meridians.

Based on Voll's principles, one can readily detect through acupuncture points and meridians the low or high energy in the body and accurately predict with the electromagnetic force of an animate or inanimate substance how these can increase or reduce energy for a specific organ or its associated pair. By being able to measure these readings on the ohmmeter, many homeopathic remedies and natural supplements can now be selected and dosages accurately calibrated for a patient at a given time of treatment. Used correctly, Voll's system can shorten the treatment of strictly monitoring the patient's subjective well-being in follow-up appointments, the Dermatron can be used to record the progress of the treatment, therefore reducing human error.

In 1953, Dr. Voll reasoned: If the assumption that each organ produces or consumes energy and that health is an energetic equilibrium which can be influenced through the respective acupuncture points are true, then it should be likewise possible with the aid of modern equipment to measure this energy and to lead it to equilibrium. Energy can be temperature, pressure, or force. It can be measured more or less precisely by various means. One form of energy, however, facilitates the measurement of the most subtle and otherwise unnoticeable changes. This energy is electricity, a phenomenon still open for definition in its ultimate sense. But, it is safe to say that it is one expression of energy.

Together with Dipl.-Ing Dr. Werner, Voll constructed a device which allows the expert to measure the slightest energy reactions and the momentary potential of an organ at the acupuncture points.

The Principle of Electro-Acupuncture According to Voll

The device Voll first used was called the DIATHERACUPUNCTURE. As recent as 1975, the DERMATRON, a more compact and transistorized instrument, has been used. The Dermatron is based on the principle that the electric potential of every organ by the application of low-level direct current can be measured precisely with the aid of a sensitive ohmmeter operated with values. The patient holds a negative electrode (made mostly of brass) while the examiner with the positive electrode locates the respective acupuncture point by using a light, mechanical pressure. These acupuncture points are located above the bone, usually in the capitulum of the joints and muscles. The patient feels no sensations from the low-alternating frequency current. The ohmmeter in the circuit indicates on a calibrated scale the magnitude or constancy of the skin resistance above the acupuncture points.

From this measurement, conclusions can be drawn as to the energetic potential of the organ, there being a defined relation between energy and resistance.

Electro-acupuncture is used in holistic diagnosis. These measurements can be used in combinations with other laboratory tests before an exact clinical diagnosis is made. This process is based on *cause* finding which cannot always be detected by conventional, orthodox means. It does not narcotize or divert, but helps by means of basic treatment which allows total health and does not lead to the *curing of symptoms.*

It is important to note that with more experience and refinement, one can by means of electro-acupuncture diagnose even parts of organs in addition to the total organs themselves. In gastric ulcers, for example, one can indicate the localization and area without having to use x-rays (roentgen) or gastroscopy.

Electro-acupuncture can verify the following states of individual organs or of the body according to the principle that health means an energetic equilibrium:

1. normal healthy energetic condition,
2. excessive energy indicating an inflammatory phase (itis),
3. too little energy indicating fatigue or degeneration (osis) of the organ,
4. an intoxication (poisoning) caused by an irradiating focus.

The Development of an Illness and Electro-Acupuncture

"How can electro-acupuncture detect illnesses in their initial stages before a considerable worsening of the body's state occurs?"

Every illness needs some time to develop. Our body is constantly exposed to all kinds of inflictions and disturbances. The body is able to cope with many irritations before cells or all compounds are damaged. We usually react with a slight uneasiness to which we attribute no major significance. Only when a larger number of cells are destroyed does our body react which clinically manifest symptoms like fever, nausea, aches, etc., and we feel sick. In any case, the smallest inflictions can cause energetic alterations.

The energetic alterations caused by every life process which, after trespassing certain limits, lead to sickness, can be detected by electro-acupuncture in the very beginnings of after-effects. The precision of measurement in electro-acupuncture is even capable of determining the day and side of the monthly ovulation in women or the changed values in the stomach shortly after ingestion which is long before the patient himself is aware of a pathological process and long before most of the clinical data can be obtained. Electro-acupuncture can indicate these conditions.

The physician can initiate counter measures to avoid severe illness or reduce it to a milder form. Similarly, beginning infectious disease can be detected by means of high measurement values long before the patient is seriously affected.

Every infection and many other disturbances of our health are not only accompanied by the classical symptoms of dolor, color, tumor, and rubor but also by an increase of the energetic potentials or an energetic barrage. The mentioned defense reactions can only build up when the energy in the body is allowed to flow freely.

The prerequisite for an optimal therapy without side- or after-effects can ideally be met by electro-acupuncture by detecting energy concentrations and controlling therapeutic measures constantly.

In degeneration processes, on the other hand, early support of perishing lesion can avoid total loss of an organ such as in cirrhosis of the liver and others.

The advantages of electro-acupuncture (early diagnosis and specific therapy without side- or after-effects), should be taken advantage of and put to use. However, electro-acupuncture should not be regarded as a competitor to established medicine but rather as a valuable means of widening it and making up for some of its shortcomings by preventive and holistic approaches.[1]

[1] H. Leonhardt, M.D., *An Introduction to Electro-Acupuncture by Voll.* Medizinisch Literarische, West Germany, 1976, pp. 17, 18

Chemotherapy and Natural Healing

It should be taken for granted that in modern medicine, the destruction of germs with the aid of chemotherapy cannot be regarded as sufficient as long as the capabilities of the various diseases could not be removed together with remnants of drugs which lead, in the long run, to iatogenic ailments so common in our time.

Basically, chemotherapy is based on the following principle: Disease is caused by a poisoning which requires an antidote. For this reason standardized quantities of pills, drugs, capsules, etc., are administered. The quantities applied are therefore, very unlikely to match the individual requirements, quite apart from the fact that every individual reacts in a different way. Not every method applied has the same results. Furthermore, some substances contain traces of other components not intended for treatment. These components may be very harmful.

In spite of these shortcomings, chemotherapy is indispensable. Additional treatment to remove residual diseases in order to avoid chemical sufferings are hard to cope with once a state of dystonia, hysteria, etc., are reached.

With the aid of electro-acupuncture, the early phases can be detected and then the development of a chronical process can be curbed. It is imperative to remove the toxins, initially hardly discernible, which orthodox medicine up to now can only trace in a few instances, since medicine's main task is restricted to the fighting of acute incidents. The intoxications are neutralized by a corresponding antitoxin and symptoms may be treated additionally with the aid of natural methods such as blaneology or physical therapy. In a simplified manner, this process can be copied in a test tube in that an agent is made to react with the respective reagent to give a neutral substance. The required dose can be quantified exactly. In somatic processes, however, several poisonous agents are mostly involved simultaneously such as toxins from bacteria, perished bacteria bodies, destroyed cells, etc. One single antitoxin usually is not enough to determine the agents involved especially since no reliable indicators are available to find out about the limits of the patient's tolerance. A great deal of expert knowledge and even intuition are required.

Homeopathy, according to Hahnemann and to Arndt-Schultz Law, is the administration of minute quantities of toxins which the organism has been exposed to, stimulating additional countermeasures of the body and thus resulting in the final elimination of the toxic disturbances. Medium doses, as often as not, are not strong enough to stimulate the body's full reactions. Excessive doses, on the other hand, can overwhelm the body's defensive mechanism.

Electro-acupuncture offers an early, simple and yet most accurate diagnosis. It is especially valuable as preventive measures in clinical medicine. Healing can be affected or strongly supported by therapeutic normalization of energetic equilibrium. Acute pain such as sciatica, cervical syndrome, etc., can be remedied immediately without side- or after-effects. And finally with undefined chronic disturbances such as migraines, asthma, gout, rheumatism, allergies, etc., electro-acupuncture can test the noxious substances whereby injections of these substances in homeopathic doses can result, in most cases, in a patient's freedom from pain.

Electro-Acupuncture Versus Chinese Acupuncture[1]

[1] H. Leonhardt, M.D., *An Introduction to Electro-Acupuncture by Voll*, Medizinisch Literarische, West Germany, 1976, pp. 17, 18

The advantages of electro-acupuncture by Voll (EAV) are:

1. EAV has a measurement device and buzzer which gives the exact acupuncture point, while Chinese acupuncture is largely based on intuition, experience and sensitivity.
2. EAV is extremely useful in clinical medicine as it can be reproduced, documented, and demonstrated on the ohmmeter. Chinese acupuncture can be verified only by pulse diagnosis which few can really master.
3. EAV can determine whether the patient is over or undertreated. Chinese acupuncture is based on the patient's reaction as to whether or not further treatment should be continued.
4. EAV can sedate or energize the acupuncture measuring point from an external means (Dermatron). A Chinese acupuncture measuring point depends on the body's own energy which supplies the acupuncture point. Consequently, these energy points depend on other sources for its energy whether it be an organ or meridian flow supplied point. If the body is low in energy, accurate results will not be produced.

5. EAV avoids the burning of moxa on the skin at the acupuncture needle site.

It is also important to note that electro-acupuncture utilizes a low alternating frequency current similar to that found in nature to produce vital body energy. This frequency range is from .8 HZ to 10 HZ. The low frequency of 1 to 3 HZ is effective in diagnosing and treating the blood and lymph disorders; of middle frequency 3 to 7 HZ in the autonomic central and peripheral nervous system; and higher frequency of 7 to 10 HZ for the treatment of organs. By using the low alternating current, 40% treatment time is saved. The purpose for the pause that follows tonification or sedation is so the body can process the stimulus to initiate the body's defensive mechanism to work and therefore, avoid exhausting or overwhelming the body's defenses.

In addition to the previous advantages, the following facts are manifest:

1. EAV can give an early diagnosis of a degenerative lesion before it is total, acute, subacute and chronic inflammation can be diagnosed and treated.
2. EAV can restore the polarization of nerves by changing the membrane potential of the cells and therefore, render the cells positive or negative. EAV can stimulate A.T.P. (adenosine triphosphate) function of a freshly injured, striated muscle.
3. EAV can tonify elastic fibers.
4. EAV can tonify smooth muscle cells in all stasis and dilations. It relieves stagnant areas in constricted drainage of lymph vessels. Therefore, all kinds of hematomas can be treated with immediate results despite the etiology.
5. EAV can reduce the inflammatory processes.
6. EAV can reduce incipient degenerative processes.

Dr. Voll has determined and verified 300 additional acupuncture points in conjunction with the traditional 800 points of the Chinese. Approximately 50 of these have dental applications. Voll was responsible in discovering acupuncture points related to general organs, sense organs, paranasal sinuses, joints, dermatomes, vertebrae, cranial nerves and the teeth. These acupuncture points were found on the classical Chinese acupuncture meridians and was not known by the Chinese. For example, it was not known before that L.I. MP-1 on the right side was related to the transverse colon. In addition to the acupuncture points founded by him, Voll did find several new meridian vessels which influence the LYMPHATIC, NERVE DEGENERATION, ALLERGY DEGENERATION, ORGAN DEGENERATION, JOINT DEGENERATION, FIBROID DEGENERATION, FAT DEGENERATION and SKIN DEGENERATION. The major control points are located in the hands and feet. Voll believes that there is less chance of error using the hands and feet rather than the ear because the acupuncture points in the ear are too close together compared to those in the hands and feet.

There are disagreements when using EAV and homeopathy as to whether the patient once treated may eat his regular diet without restrictions. The patient can get well with EAV and homeopathic remedies, but these dysfunctions will eventually surface again, especially if those ingested chemicals contributed to the original cause. Therefore, it is my belief that an optimal diet (balancing effect of foods and supplements) along with a controlled exercise program are necessary requirements in the *preservation of aging tissues and the equilibrium of the body's energies.* Furthermore, ridding the body of degenerative producing stimuli such as vaccination and insecticide poisons can propagate the demise of the body's recuperative powers. In short, EAV offers a new dimension in the diagnosis, prevention and ultimate cure of these factors.

NOTES

DIAGNOSTIC EVALUATION OF THE MEASUREMENT CRITERIA

The Dermatron

The DERMATRON is an instrument which precisely measures the skin resistance above the acupuncture point. It measures tissues whose energy potential can be converted into a readable measurement on a calibrated ohmmeter. One is then able to detect fatigue, degeneration or low energy, inflammation or high energy, and irritation which is tolerable to the body tissue providing it is stable. So when measuring the acupuncture points of the body, a stable measurement value remains constant over the entire measurement. Measurement values reaching their maximum peak very slowly without an indicator drop can be interpreted as an organic fatigue in its initial stage of insufficiency. In measuring the value of the acupuncture points, the most important criterion Voll found is the indicator drop (ID). This means that the point does not have a stable value because the value drops down from a higher to a lower value during the same measurement. You have to wait until the indicator stops dropping and keeps its value at a stable stage.

The Indicator Drop

Voll explains an indicator drop: In functional disturbed organs, the bioelectric resistance to the measurement current is decreased and the organ is not able to maintain a constant resistance to the intruding current. The decrease in bioelectric efficiency is revealed by an indicator drop which manifests itself in the state of equilibrium between stimulation by the measurement current and the reactive capability of the organ. The difference between the maximum labile and the minimum stabile values require differential evaluation. As a rule, the indicator drop after reaching its maximum value occurs within 1-3 seconds. In a retarded indicator drop indicative of an incipient functional disturbance, the period of 3 seconds may be exceeded such as in a beginning odontogenic focal disturbances measurable on one of the 6 maxillary and mandibular measurement points. The interval for the indicator drop from its initial maximum value to its final minimum value depends on the intensity and scope of the pathological process in the organ measured.

Internal for the Indicator drop:

Above 50 values .... 10 to 20 seconds
Value drops to 30 .... 20 to 30 seconds
Value drops to 20 or less .... 30 to 60 seconds
(in cases of cancer)

Pathological Anatomic Evaluation of the Measurement Values[2]

[2] Reinhold Voll, M.D., "Twenty Years of Electro-Acupuncture Diagnosis in Germany A Progress Report." American Journal of Acupuncture, March 1975, pp. 6, 7

100-92 Total inflammation — total itis, whole organ involved.

88-82 Partial inflammation — partial itis, portion of the organ is inflamed as in a decreasing organ inflammation or a fascial inflammation of the organ.

80-66 Cumulative irritations, approaching inflammation. Treatment necessary.

The latter leads to a premorbid situation:

65-52 Irritations in the physiological area — no treatment is necessary if there is no indicator drop.

50 Ideal value for the harmotonic state or normal energy.

48-40 Incipient degeneration — beginning — ose.

38-30 Advanced degeneration — advanced — ose.

28-20 Considerable degeneration — final state of — ose.

Less than 20— Degeneration in the final stages, cancer.

Less than 10 — Before death.

According to Voll, try to bring the values to 50 which will protect the patient against multiple irritation of the work day without vegetative or organic stray reactions.

Degenerative situations are characterized by insufficient energy production and by metabolic depression of cellular functions resulting in cellular dystrophy.

An indicator drop is the most important criteria for EAV. In diagnosis, one should always deter mine the indicator drops for the patient and enter them on his records. It is also important to rate the speed of rise of the indicator needle, the maximum height of the needle and the speed and time of the drop.

If an indicator drop is present in more than 10 units, then an acute disturbance in that respective organ is indicated and immediate treatment must begin.

If the indicator drop is indicated on 6 terminal points on the hand or foot, then a field of disturbances most likely in the colon area is involved.

If an indicator drop is experienced on the circulation MP-9 (arteries), lymph MP-1,2 (palatine tonsil and dental point), endocrine control measurement point, and spleen MP-1, then there is a humoral or fluid imbalance in the body. The deep cervical lymph nodes T.W. 16a can also be measured for humoral disturbances.

When you have a total indicator drop of 6 points on both hands only, then an allergenic reaction is indicated.

A total of 12 indicator drops on one side of the body, 6 on the hand and 6 on the foot can point to a neural disturbance. For example, the hand may have an ID on the terminal points on heart, endocrine, circulation, large intestine, small intestine and lung meridian while the foot may have an ID on the pancreas, liver, stomach, gallbladder, kidney and urinary bladder meridians.

A combination of 12 ID on both hands and 6 ID on one foot will indicate a combination of neural allergenic reactions.

If indicator measurements reach a high of 90 with a minimal drop on 40, this indicates an inflammatory stage with a premorbid or incipient degeneration of the organ.

NOTES

Other combinations in the maximum-minimum ranges may exist as follows:

Pathological Anatomic Evaluation of the Indicator Drop[3]

[3] Reinhold Voll, M.D., "Twenty Years of Electro-Acupuncture Diagnosis in Germany A Progress Report." American Journal of Acupuncture, March 1975, pp. 6, 7

ID: INDICATOR DROP *manifests destruction of parenchyma cells. It occurs in all sorts of inflammation except the serous inflammation.*

ID 92 to 82 Total inflammation with dead cells. Dx. infectious organic inflammation — affected.

ID 88 to 82 Partial "itis" with cellular destruction. Dx. focus, decreasing organic inflammation with partial inflammation.

ID 74 to 70 Minor incipient degenerative process in a non-inflamed organ.

ID 90 to 44 At the MP heart muscle (Heart-6) bilaterally. Dx. acute inflammatory myocarditis against a background of myocardosis.

ID 88 to 20 At the MP left bronchus (Lung-10). Dx. partial "itis" in a bronchocarcinoma.

ID 94 to 46 At the MP hepatic cell. Dx. acute hepatitis with a violent course.

ID 86 to 52 At MP hepatic cell. Dx. hepatitis in regression. Still has extensive area of insular inflammation.

In case of chronic bronchitis, which does not respond to any kind of treatment, a value of 88 with indicator drop (88/78 or less) may be found on one side. On the other side the control measurement point of the lung may be 84/22 (slow) which means on that side a cancer can be expected.

THE DERMATRON

The Instrument and Its Uses

The DERMATRON has come into its use for EAV diagnosis for physicians and dentists. Compared to its predecessor, the K & F Diatheracupuncteur developed in 1953 by Voll, the DERMATRON is a much lighter transistorized instrument with the same electrophysical parameters as the vacuum tube instrument. The DERMATRON is able to charge the acupuncture points with direct current in the order of 8-10 microamperes and approximately 1 volt. This amounts to a measurement of the resistance of the skin above the acupuncture point. This instrument is calibrated from "0-100" and is marked with the number 50 at the central position indicating that the organ or part of the organ associated with the acupuncture points is free of pathological problems.

It takes only a few seconds to diagnose a specific acupuncture point with this machine. It enables the operator to make a differential diagnosis by comparing several reference points on the depressions and elevations of bone, or over interarticum spaces, above furrows in joint cartilages and in certain muscles. By scanning a topographic position of an acupuncture point the doctor is able to determine whether the specific acupuncture point is measured at the precise center. This has the advantage of the classical acupuncture technique. Measurement of the progress, using low alternating frequency current therapy and homeopathic remedies, can be instituted into a disciplined treatment routine. In addition to using medications, the therapeutic process of radiation, hydrotherapy, hot baths, special gymnastics, massages, etc., can be measured. The progress can be measured exactly at the appropriate points. An unclear influencing field of disturbances can be diagnosed as to its effect on the foci of infection. Undetermined causal weak links which may alter the course of treatment can be established. Related organs, muscle, joints, vertebrae, nervous system, lymphatics, vascular and humoral can be compared as conflicting alterations to its total effect on the total modality of cure. By energizing (tonifying) or sedating (relaxing) of the tissues we can decrease the degenerative and inflammatory process within the body.

Other advantages of this instrument is the feature of the absence of parasitic radiation from outside sources. The Dermatron is operated by a rechargeable battery which is used only when in operation. It takes 10 hours to charge and to maintain an active current within the instrument so that a consistent, repeatable reading can be performed. The soundswitch for the acoustic electro-acupuncture enables the operator to determine whether he is on the middle of the point itself. The variopit is a gold metallic baton which incorporates a light and sound system to locate without any pressure, the point of measurement.

Frequency in HZ and intensity in electricity* can be adjusted to the specific condition of the patient whether it be a vascular, lymphatic, neural or muscular disturbance. A quick diagnosis can be made as to what quadrant of the body (head, left or right trunk and feet) is lacking energy or is imbalanced with the rest of the body.

This enables the doctor to quickly evaluate where the foci of disturbance may be. Another added feature is that it can be automatically regulated during treatment, enabling the patient to read the diagnostic and therapy values as shown on the ohmmeters.

Various accessories such as foot plates, rectal and vaginal electrodes, roller electrodes, sheet electrodes, mini-electrodes can be utilized for the various treatment modality. An external ohmmeter can be attached to the Dermatron for teaching purposes.

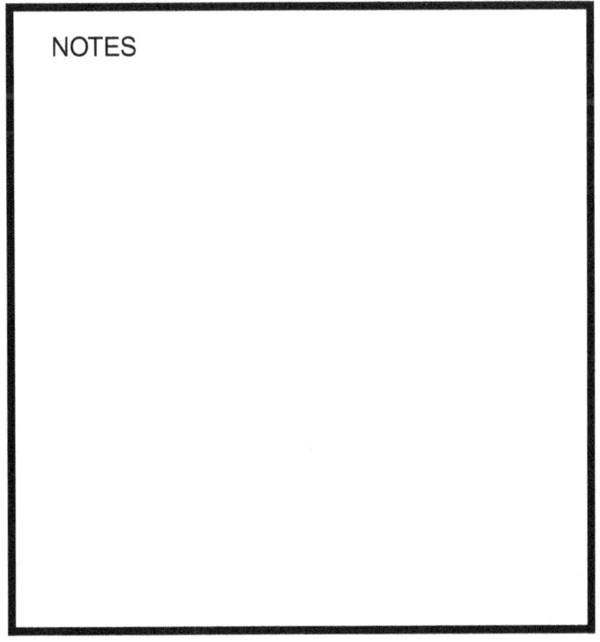

The Dermatron using EAV enables the professional to confirm diagnostic methods and monitor therapeutic progress as well as failures. This method is useful in cardiology, angiology, pulmonology, gastroenterology, hepatology, urology, gynecology, otorhinolaryngology, endocrinology, orthopedics, dermatology, neurology, dentistry and ophthalmology.

EAV makes it possible to have an early diagnosis and consequently accomplish preventive therapy. One must keep in mind that x-ray diagnosis is not an early but a late stage diagnosis. Laboratory diagnostic methods are only employed when the disease has reached a certain level. It is the responsibility of the doctor to make an early diagnosis so as to reverse this process by appropriate measures before this disease requires surgery for repairs. It must be borne in mind that these preventive measures may not show clinically but already show certain levels of illnesses.

Application of the Rectal Electrode in Men

1. For all diseases of the urinary bladder.
2. For all diseases of the prostate.
3. For all diseases of the seminal vesicle.
4. For all diseases of the seminal vesicle's terminal portion. In cases one to four (1-4) place sheet electrode as counter-electrode over the symphysis urinary bladder region. It is necessary to lubricate the rectal electrode.
5. For diseases of the anal canal and anal fissures. It is necessary to lubricate the rectal electrode.
6. For diseases of the rectum, it is useful to grease the rectal electrode with a hemorrhoidal ointment. In cases five to six (5-6) the counter - electrode should be placed over the lower sacral bone and the coccyx.
7. For diseases of the sacral bone and the coccyx, place the counter-electrode over the sacral bone and the coccyx.
8. For diseases of the hip joint, place sheet electrode as counter-electrode over the anterior lower inguinal ligament when pain is located there, or over the trochanter region which is done more frequently.
9. For kidney stones in the ureter in front of the bladder.

Application of the Rectal and Vaginal Electrode in Women Fig. 600

1. For inflammatory diseases of the uterus and and its adjacent regions, the vaginal electrode is useful. The vaginal electrode has to touch the portio. Place the sheet electrode as a counter-electrode over the small of the back.
2. For diseases of the anal canal, hemorrhoids and anal fissures, the rectal electrode is used. Place the counter-electrode over the sacral bone and the coccyx.
3. For diseases of the rectum (see under item 6 in men).
4. For diseases of the sacral bone and the coccyx, use the rectal electrode as under item 7 in men.
5. For diseases of the sacroiliac joint, use the sheet electrode as a positive electrode over the joint and the rectal electrode as counter-electrode.

Fig. 600 — **Vaginal Electrode**

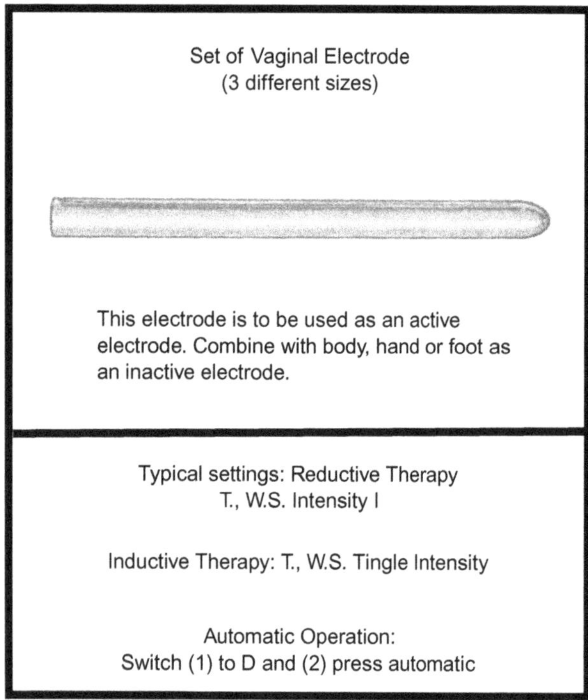

Set of Vaginal Electrode
(3 different sizes)
This electrode is to be used as an active electrode. Combine with body, hand or foot as an inactive electrode.
Typical settings: Reductive Therapy
T., W.S. Intensity I
Inductive Therapy: T., W.S. Tingle Intensity
Automatic Operation:
Switch (1) to D and (2) press automatic

6. For diseases of the hip joint, use the vaginal electrode and the sheet electrode as a counter-electrode as under item 8 in men.
7. For diseases of the ovaries, place the counter-electrode over the hypogastrium in the ovary region and use the vaginal electrode.
8. For vaginitis, use the vaginal electrode and rectal electrode as counter-electrode or sheet electrode over the urinary bladder region.
9. For diseases of the urinary bladder, use the vaginal electrode and sheet as counter electrode over and below the symphysis.
10. For diseases of the urethra, use vaginal electrode and sheet electrode as counter-electrode over and below the symphysis.
11. For intended pregnancy, use the vaginal electrode and one counter-electrode each on the left and right ovary.
12. For frigidity, use vaginal electrode and one counter-electrode each on the gonad measurement points on the medial side of the left and right thigh in the lower angle of Scarpa's triangle.
13. For thrombophlebitis in the anterior portion of the pelvis, use the vaginal electrode and counter-electrode over the left and right hypogastrium. For thrombophlebitis in the posterior portion of the pelvis, use the sheet electrode as counter-electrode over the sacral bone.

Application of the Roller Electrode Fig 601

1. For all lymphatic stasis as an accompanying therapy after operations, for example, in the mouth and the jaws (after difficult tooth extractions).
2. For elephantiasis and lymphatic stasis in the lower leg.
3. For after-treatment in gearing the energy circulation to painful and energy deficient areas.
4. For electrical moxibustion treatment, use roller electrode as counter-electrode in periostitis, such as in epicondylitis of the humerus, calcaneus spur, etc.
5. For all chronic inflammations of nerves within the extent of the inflamed nerve, such as in trigeminal neuralgia, facial paresis, etc.

Fig. 601 — **B1 — Polar Roller Electrode**

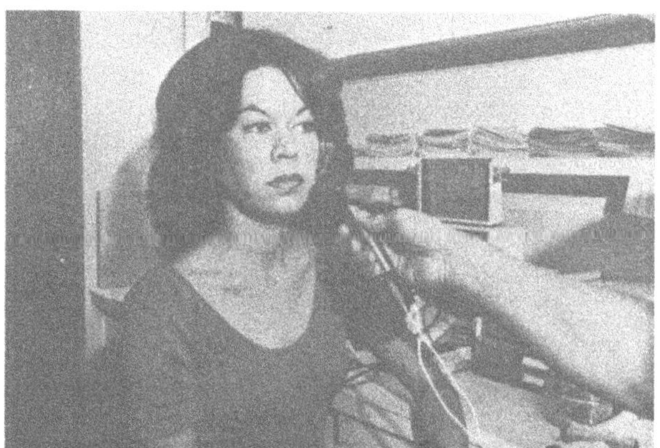

6. For all kinds of myalgias and myogeloses. Apply the roller until softening of the myalgia and reddening of the skin result, such as on both sides of the vertebral skin in acute lumbago or chronic lumbalgia. In torticollis, the roller is applied on the sternocleidomastoid muscle.
7. General roller electrode treatment as an additional treatment after flooding the joints by the sheet electrode.
8. Roller electrode treatment following contusion of joints or distortion of joints after previous basic treatment on hands or feet in addition to the treatment of the points relating to the impaired joints.

Fig. 602 — **Diagram for EAV Dermatron Connection**

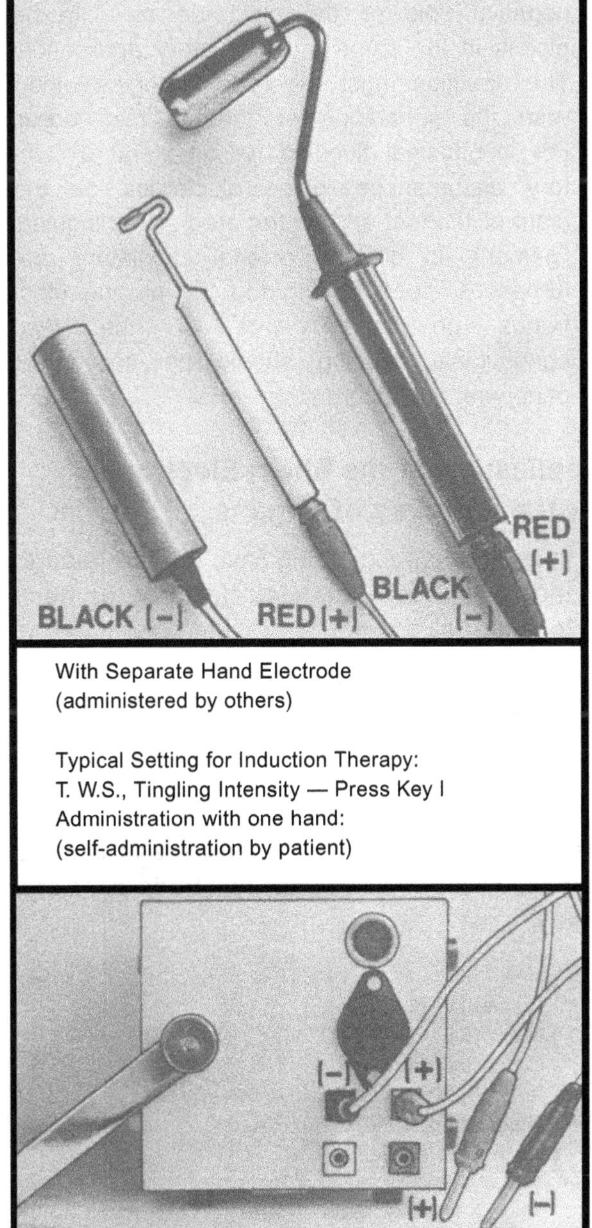

Indication for the Mini-Roller Electrode

To be applied in the oral cavity, in gingivitis, over inflamed gingivae pockets, in areas around partially impacted teeth. Fig. 603

Fig. 603 — **Miniroller used for Gum Treatment can be Autoclaved**
Setting: Tingle Intensity — T., W.S. Tingle
Basic Rule: *Active* electrode on area to be treated

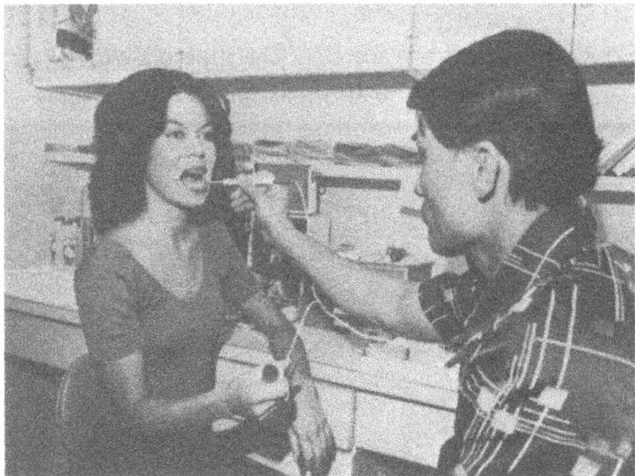

Indication for the Foot Electrode

For inflamed flat foot and pes valgus, place the counter-electrode on the dorsum of the foot.

Indication for the Ear Electrode

For otitis externa and for furunculosis of the external auditory canal, use the counter-electrode over the zygomatic arch close to the ear.

Application of the Sheet Electrode

1. Place the sheet electrode like a short wave electrode.
   a. Tranverse flooding of arthritic/arthrotic joints in hydrarthrosis, hemarthrosis and in hematomas.
   b. Longitudinal flooding of portions of the extremities in disturbances or arterial circulation and venous stasis.

Fig. 604 — **Diagram for EAV Dermatron with Sheet Electrodes**

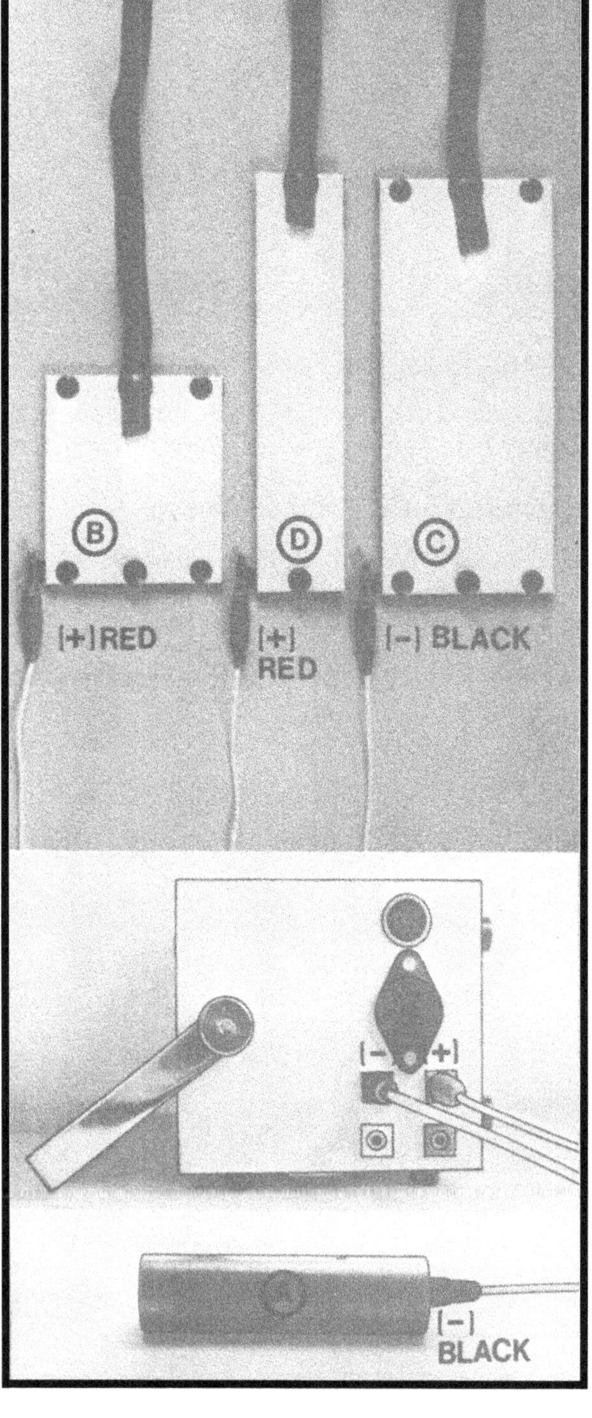

Special Indications

1. Flooding of organ portions in scar (keloid) formation, such as on the hand: Dupuytren's Disease, use inactive electrode on the palm and sheet electrode on the dorsum of the hand, or, for example, on the penis in enduratio penis plastica, place one small sheet electrode each on the lower and upper side of the penis.
2. Flooding after fractures. Electrodes are being placed proximally and distally to the plaster cast in order to accelerate callus formation. Transverse flooding of the joint following contusion or torsion to intensity resorption of the hematoma.
3. Longitudinal flooding of the extremity in thrombophlebitis. Note that the positive and the negative pole of the electrode have to be placed in the same order in every application: The direction must never be changed, otherwise the separation of thrombi may occur. For longitudinal flooding for unilateral circulatory disturbances, place electrodes on the plant of the foot and on the area of the inguinal ligament. In bilateral arterial circulatory disturbances, flood foot to foot by placing electrodes on both plants of the feet. Longitudinal flooding should be applied in peripheral neuralgias.

Application of the Sheet Electrodes for the Flooding of Organs

1. In headaches extending from the forehead to the nape, use one sheet electrode on each location.
2. In lateral headache, use lateral flooding. Place one electrode above the ear.

Myalgias

In myalgia of the masseter muscle, place sheet electrode on the masseter muscle and use the vaginal electrode as counter-electrode in the oral cavity.

Ⓐ HAND ELECTRODE INACTIVE
Connection: BLACK (—)
Ⓑ BODY ELECTRODE ACTIVE
Connection: RED (+)
Ⓒ "LARGE" BODY ELECTRODE INACTIVE
Connection: BLACK (—)
Ⓓ "SMALL" BODY ELECTRODE ACTIVE
Typical setting for Inductive Therapy:
Tingle— Intensity, T., W.S.
Basic Rule: ACTIVE Electrode on Area to be Treated

NOTES

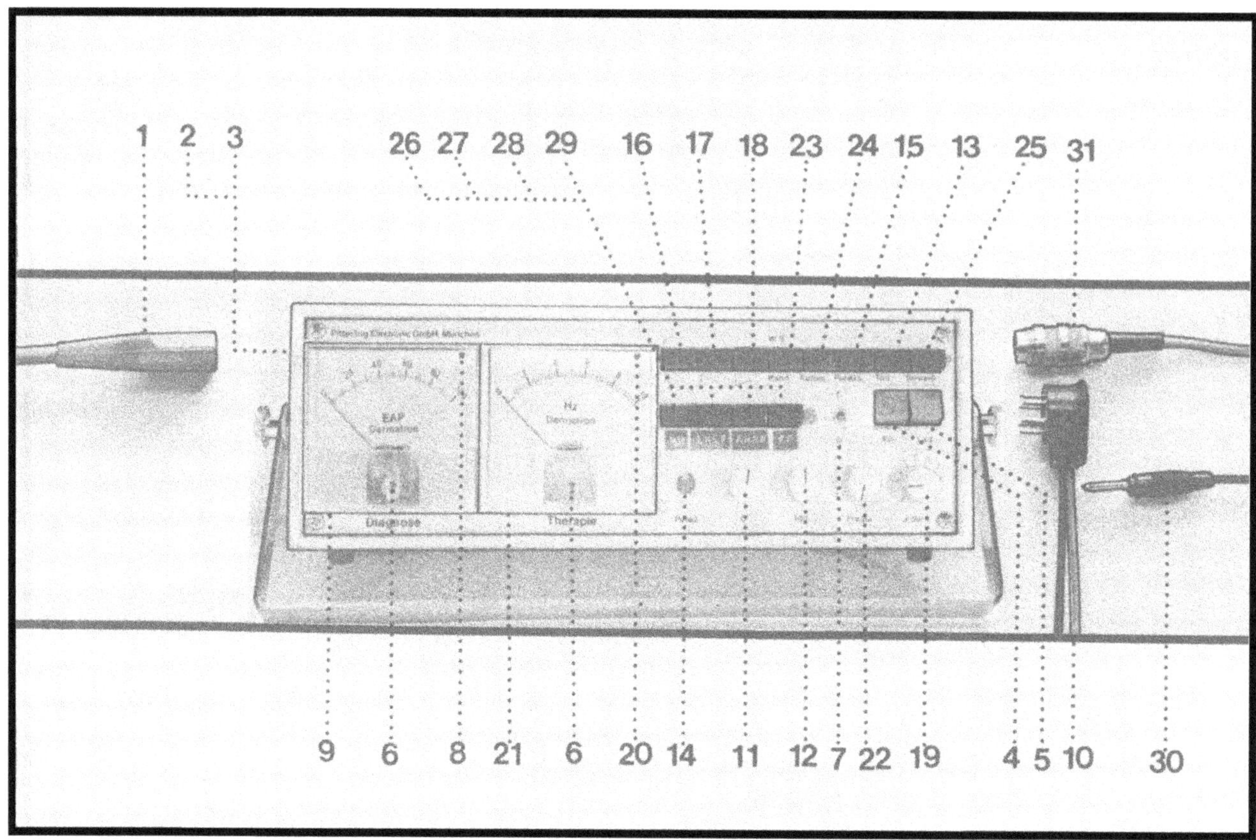

Fig 605 — **EAV Dermatron**

OPERATING INSTRUCTIONS FOR EAV DERMATRON Fig. 605

1. .... Net cable.
2. .... Net socket, on left lateral part.
3. .... Main fuse.

4 .... Main ON/OFF switch with control lamp green **(ON)**.

5. .... Charge switch with control lamp red **(CHARGE)**.
6. .... ZERO-correction.
7. .... Tumbler switch diagnosis/therapy **(D/T)**.
8. .... Control lamp for diagnosis.
9. .... Visual indicator for diagnosis and point research.
10. .... Socket for measuring cable **(SIX-POLE SOCKET)**.
11. .... Zero-calibration for diagnosis **(0)**.
12. .... 100-calibration for diagnosis **(100)**.
13. .... Sound switch for acoustic electro-acupuncture.
14. .... Sensitivity regulator for point-research-part.
15. .... Change-over switch from diagnosis to point research.
16. .... Key depressed:
17. .... Therapy switch, key depressed: positive.
18. .... Therapy switch, key depressed: negative.
19. .... Intensity regulator **(INTENS.)**.
20. .... Control lamp for therapy.

21. ....Indicator instrument for therapy frequency.
22. ....Regulator for firm frequency setting **(FREQU.).**
23. ....Change-over switch from wave-swinging.
24. ....Automatic switch-over from diagnosis to therapy **(AUTOM.)**.
25. ....Change-over switch for stylus control from therapy to writing.
26. .... **Key I** pushed in: hand/hand.
27. ....4-Quadrant selectors ... **Key II** pushed in: left hand/left foot.
28. .... **Key III** pushed in: right hand/right foot.
29. .... **Key IV** pushed in: foot/foot.
30. ....Sockets for 4-Quadrant-electrodes **(DISTINGUISHING COLOR MARK):** Fig. 606

(BLACK) = left hand
(RED) = right hand
(GREEN) = right foot
(YELLOW) = left foot

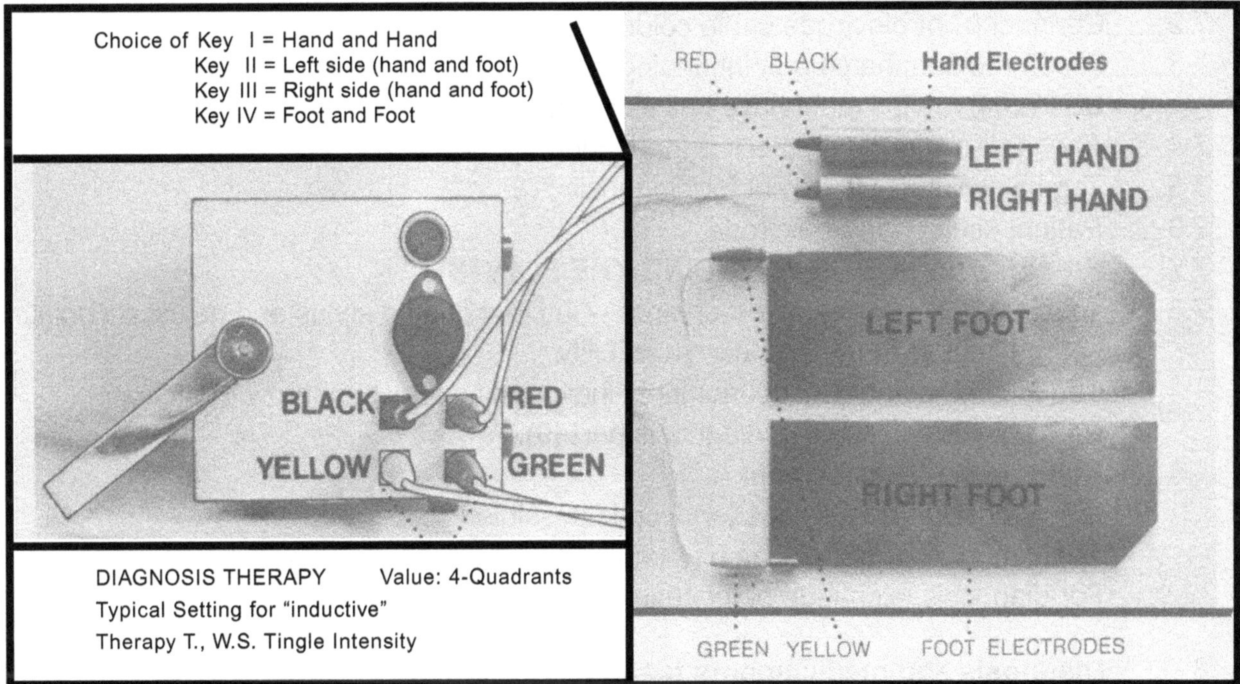

Fig. 606 — **Diagram to Connect the Hand and Foot Electrodes**

31. ....Socket for writing set.

5. ....**Functioning test**

Basic setting as under pos. **3.1** or **4.1.**

5.1 ....Tumbler switch **(7)** depress for diagnosis **"D."** Control lamp **(8)** shines in instrument of diagnosis **(9).**

5.2 ....Connect measurement cable. Put six-pole connector into outlet 10 on right hand side of housing.

5.3 ....Connect measurement stylus on cable **(BAYONET CONNECTION).**

5.4 ....Screw on top of stylus measurement-cones according to your choice **(ELECTRODE ON STYLUS RED = POSITIVE).**

5.5 ....Connect hand-electrode with banana plug **(BLACK = NEGATIVE)**.

6. -------- **Calibration "0" and "100"**
Basic setting as under pos. **3.1 or 4.1.**

6.1 -------- Calibrate knife edge pointer **(9)** into "0"-position with "0"-knob **(11)** by turning knob either right or left.

6.2 -------- Bring together by touching stylus electrode with hand-electrode for short circuit. Calibrate for "100" on instrument indicator **(9)** by turning calibration knob "100" **(12)** either right or left.
Note: After heavy mechanical stress under transport conditions it might be necessary to adjust both indicator instruments **(DIAGNOSIS AND THERAPY)** by turning position 6 with a screw driver. **(INDICATOR IN "OPPOSITION.)**
Set has been adjusted in factory.

7. -------- **Finding the points**
Basic setting as under pos. **3.1** or **4.1.**
The cable, necessary for finding the points, is marked with a red point on plug.

7.1 -------- Take off measuring cable.

7.2 -------- Connect point electrode cable color mark on six-pole plug.

7.3 -------- Fix on red banana plug point finding stylus **(STYLUS WITHOUT THERAPY BUTTON)**. Stylus must have ball electrode.

7.4 -------- Fix hand-electrode on black banana plug.

7.5 -------- Toggle-switch **(7)** to be set for diagnosis **"D."**

7.6 -------- Patient keeps hand-electrode.

7.7 -------- Press key 15 **(KEY FOR FINDING THE POINTS).**

7.8 -------- Touch skin of patient in search area with point finding stylus and adjust on point search knob **(14)** the indicator sensibility.
The located point of acupuncture is indicated by maximal throw of indicator (VALUE 100) on scale in diagnosis part **(9).**
Comparable Measurement.
In this position only point searching is possible.
The valuation of points can neither be measured nor determined.
For diagnosis exchange point search cable with measurement cable.

8. -------- **Diagnosis and medicaments testing**
82 = standard for hand-foot/foot-foot **(ROUGH MEASUREMENT).**
50 = standard when point mensuration.
Basic setting as under pos. **3.1** or **4.1.**

Functioning test

a. Basic setting as under pos. **3.1** or **4.1.**
b. Tumbler switch **(7)** depress for diagnosis **"D."** Control lymph **(8)** shines in instrument of diagnosis **(9)**.
c. Connect measurement cable. Put six-pole connector into outlet on right hand side of housing.
d. Connect measurement stylus on cable **(BAYONET CONNECTION).**
e. Screw on top of stylus measurement-cones according to your choice **(ELECTRODE ON STYLUS RED = POSITIVE).**
f. Connect hand-electrode with banana plug **(BLACK = NEGATIVE).**

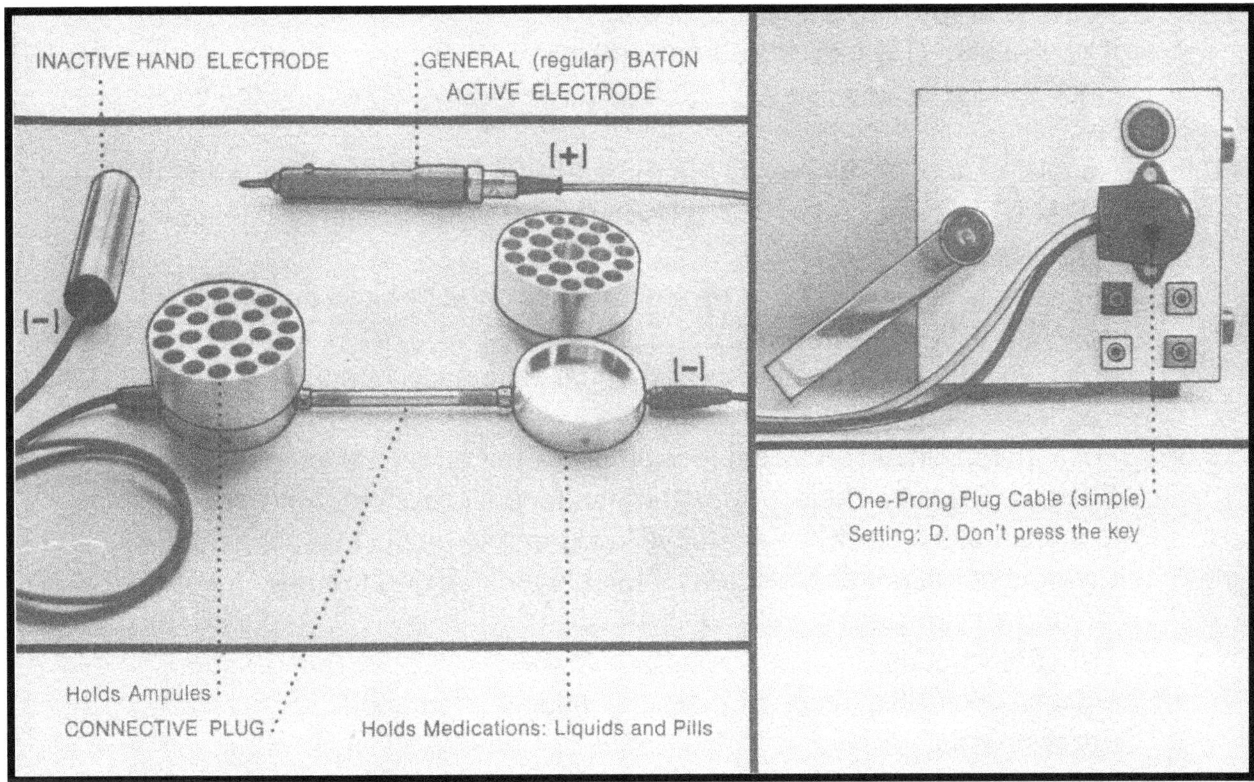

Fig. 607 — **Diagram of Connection of Honeycomb (holds medication) to Electrodes from the Dermatron**

8.1 .... Push in key **"TON" (13).**
Note: Key **(15)** = point finder key; should not be pushed in, since the whole set would be blocked.
In this position diagnosis and testing of medicaments can be made.

8.2 .... Measurement of 4-quadrants:

8.3 .... With above setting connect quadrant-cables **(BLACK/RED/YELLOW/GREEN)** on the lateral leading off **(30).**

8.4 .... Fixation of hand-electrodes on banana plugs **BLACK/RED.**

8.5 .... Fixation of foot-electrodes on banana plugs **YELLOW/GREEN.**

8.6 .... Key I **(26)** pressed in = hand-hand = **BLACK,** left hand/**RED,** right hand.
Key II **(27)** pressed in = left hand = **BLACK,** left foot = **YELLOW.**
Key III **(28)** pressed in = right hand = RED, right foot = **GREEN.**
Key IV **(29)** pressed in = foot-foot = left foot = **YELLOW**
right foot = **GREEN.**

9. .... **Automatic operation**
(Automatic switching from therapy to diagnostic part in basic therapy.) Only significant when value 82 should be attained hand-hand/foot-foot.
Basic setting as under position **3.1 (4.1)** and therapy position **10** with pos. **10.4.**

9.1 .... Push key "Automatic" **(24).**

9.2 .... Press down tumbler switch **(7)** into diagnosis position **"D"** control lights **8** and **20** light up reciprocally.

10. .... **Therapy**
Basic setting as pos. **3.1 or 4.1.**

10.1........ **Point-Therapy** See pos. **5.1** until **5.5.**
Key "Punkts." **(15)** may not be pressed in.

10.2........ Choose kind of impulse .... by depressing the corresponding key.

10.3........ Regulate knob 19 for intensity to generate **(WEAKEN)** ....: Intensity **0, 5 (SCALE)** to build up **(STRENGTHEN)** ....prickle intensity approximately 3-5 **(SCALE).**

10.4........ "WS" key **(23)** not pushed in = automatic change of biofrequencies **(RANGE 0, 9 — 10 CYCLES).**
"WS" key **(23)** when pushed in = manual setting for a frequency. Regulate with frequency adjuster **(22).**

10.5........ Point therapy in action by depressing press-button on measurement stylus.

10.6........ **Surface Therapy** (therapy with great surface electrodes).
Quadrant cable black/red and/or yellow/green to be put into connections.

10.7........ Connect corresponding electrode suitable for intended therapy:
hand-electrodes
foot-electrodes
body-electrodes (made of elastic, conducting material)
Roller unipolar
Roller bipolar
Vaginal electrode
Rectal electrode, etc.
Fundamental rule: Active electrode **(RED OR GREEN)** to be placed on spot where treatment is necessary. Inactive electrode as counter-electrode yellow or black.

10.8........ Push either key I, II, III, IV according to desired leading off. See pos. **8.6.**

10.9........ See pos. **10.2** and **10.4.**

10.9.1 ....Push tumbler switch (7) topwards into **"T"** position (THERAPY) control lamp lights up.

10.9.2 ....Push either key I, II, III, IV according to desired leading off. See pos. **8.6.**

10.9.2 ....Regulate knob for intensity **(19).** See pos. **10.3.**
.... = Abbau
.... = Aufbau
.... = Pseudoaufbau
Pseudoaufbau is applied, for instance, in case of a collapse to supply patient with high energy.
For example, collapse situation shows on indicator instrument.
Approx. value 40.
With key ....(Pseudoaufbau) value increases up to value 70 on indicator instrument.
Value diminishes again and stabilizes as far as 80.

11. .... **Peripheral equipment** Connection of writing set on EAV-DERMATRON.

11.1........ Put connection plug in measurement socket **(31).**

11.2 .... Push key "Schreib" **(25).**

11.3........ With press-button on stylus-electrode writing set can be put into action.

THERAPEUTIC PART OF THE DERMATRON

Current characteristics can be used to achieve therapy without resorting to medication.

This therapy is based on energetic concepts where you add or subtract electric balances into the body at specific body organs or sites that may be experiencing pain.

FLOODING

Flooding is useful for articular complaints. Use one electrode on one side of the body and the other on the opposite side. Use the intensity just barely tolerable on the pain area of the patient. Flood for 5 minutes and you may get a result; stop the treatment. Add another 2 to 5 minutes and get rid of the pain in addition to the swelling. Use alternating current with maximum intensity. Use maximum frequency 10 HZ because the treatment goes faster.

For flooding in the head, use a lesser frequency in the range of 6 HZ because the head cannot tolerate high frequencies. Use the WS, waveswing, although it takes longer if you are unsure of the frequency required. WS will sweep and find the specific frequency which is covered by the movement of the indicator and thus will influence the disturbed area specifically.

Flooding can be used on the ankle joint, knee joint, elbow, shoulder, wrist joint and ileo-sacral joint. In addition to the joints, you can treat the lower abdominals, pain associated with any kind of irregular organ functions especially in irregular menstruation, genital or urinary organs or chronic prostatics. For example, the flooding technique is advantageous with chronic urinary bladder inflammation which is hard to cope with antibiotics. For women, use vaginal electrode and the counter-electrode on the pubis. It can, in some instances, remove the original cause such as in the cystics of the ovaries.

Flooding will work only in reactive ranges and not when the pathology has gotten to a stage where it is hard to tackle with these energetic means. A surgeon is needed when malignancies set in.

Flooding can be used instead of medications, but it is time consuming and may take as much as 6 weeks. On stubborn conditions, the patient may not be immediately aware of any changes. After the first or second week, a change will take place and he will be encouraged to being further treated.

Flooding improves the lymphatic drainage. As the transportation of poison is better, the circulation of the lymph is improved. By flooding, the stasis is treated. Flooding will take care of organic tissue. The bacteria can no longer take advantage of the situation. Flooding can take care of fibroid, vascular and lymphatic disturbances.

Flooding is a more local or symptomatic treat**ment.** It is better to get rid of the primary foci of disturbances, a constant one, rather than the remote one. Head and jaw area, treat with low intensity and frequency. Avoid any flashing or flickering of the eyes, which indicates that the intensity is too high. For tinnitus, especially in small children, apply the active electrode on the back of the ear and the inactive electrode on the front of the ear. This will improve the lymphatic and vascular situation, and the ear pains will suddenly go away.

Flooding is good for local condition of rhinitis and sinusitis. Place electrodes on the area to relieve the stasis and the assembly of the mucus and lymph may drain properly. However, this would not take care of the underlying situation.

Flooding is good for post extractions to reduce swelling.

Flooding will not remove toxins; nosode treatment will. It is the only means of stimulating the tissue to respond. When the stimulus is not high enough to reach the threshold, there will be no response, no reaction. Homeopathy lowers the threshold and allows the stimulus to get through.

Flooding may restore some measures of sight and hearing in the senile and deaf.

In generalized arthritis, flooding will relieve the pain for a short time. This is a systemic disease rather than a localized disease. For isolated articular pains, mostly the big toe joint, flooding is ideal for short intervals. For treating local pains, flood first when there is no relief. Decrease the intensity and switch to a positive characteristic to sedate it. In inflammatory processes, add energy because inflammation is a response of the body. When you add energy from the outside, the body does not need to be in an inflammatory state itself. When treating localized areas of pain that are chronic and not acute, use flooding and balance the meridians.

However, the best treatment is to treat the organs since they take care of the entire body. The organs take care of the growth processes, healing, metabolic changes and catabolic changes.

Flooding can give pain relief but does not cure the underlying cause.

Flooding is good for vertebral spine pain. Place the electrode next to the spine and not on it.

In thrombophlebitis in the leg, flooding is useful to take care of an acute event. Make sure you place the electrodes on the distal part and the proximal part. Keep this in order and not reverse the active or inactive electrodes in following appointments or it will cause thrombus which may get loose and plug up some vessels elsewhere ending up in an embolism.

CROSS HATCHING

CROSS HATCHING is a useful technique in treating muscle spasms, strains, tendon and ligament injuries. The Dermatron is turned on to its highest frequency, **10 HZ** and **intensity 10.**

The first energy button is depressed as well as the **HH** button. This maximum frequency and intensity is applied to the trigger areas of pain.

For example: When treating a muscle spasm in the back such as the sacrospinalis, place the grounding brass electrode (black cord) of the Dermatron on the spine blocking the nerve reflexes from the trigger area of the muscle to the spine. The red electrode is then applied on the trigger area of the muscle in a scratching pattern, and thus the name CROSS HATCHING.

This pattern is done quickly as this procedure is discomforting. The treated muscle undergoes a massive contraction. Muscle fatigue follows and the toxic lactic acid is flushed through the lymphatic vessels. When the current is removed from the muscle, the muscles then return to their physiological resting length. Pain in the muscle is reduced and in many cases completely diminished. The therapy is continued when the skin over the muscle turns red and the pain has diminished.

MASSETER MUSCLE SPASM

1. Setting: 10 HZ, 10 INTENSITY, first energy button depressed, HH button depressed.
2. Place BRASS GROUNDING ELECTRODE (NEGATIVE BLACK) above the zygomatic bone. This is near the origin of the masseter muscles.
3. The POSITIVE RED ELECTRODE is applied to the gogli tendons in a cross hatching pattern.
4. Repeat this CROSS HATCHING method on the lower jaw on the area where the masseter muscle joins the lower external border of the jaw.
5. Keep the NEGATIVE BLACK ELECTRODE on the lower jaw and cross hatch the spindle cells on the belly of the muscles.

TINNITUS

1. Place the NEGATIVE ELECTRODE in front of the ear.
2. CROSS HATCH behind the ear over acupuncture points TW-17 MIDDLE EAR and TW-18 INTERNAL EAR.

LYMPHATIC STASIS

1. Place the NEGATIVE ELECTRODE on the mesial of the sternocleidomastoid muscles at the angle of the jaw.
2. The deep cervical lymph nodes **TW-16a** is on the center of this sternocleidomastoid muscle.
3. CROSS HATCH the deep cervical lymph node which will cause the toxins from the eye, ear and teeth to drain.

CARPAL TUNNEL SYNDROME & TARSAL TUNNEL SYNDROME

1. Place the NEGATIVE ELECTRODE between the heart and the area treated on the arm or leg.
2. CROSS HATCH with the POSITIVE ELECTRODE on the tendon until there is relief from the pain.

CALCANEOUS SPUR

1. Place the NEGATIVE ELECTRODE below the ankle.
2. CROSS HATCH the calcaneous spur with the POSITIVE ELECTRODE.
3. Repeat this treatment until the pain disappears.

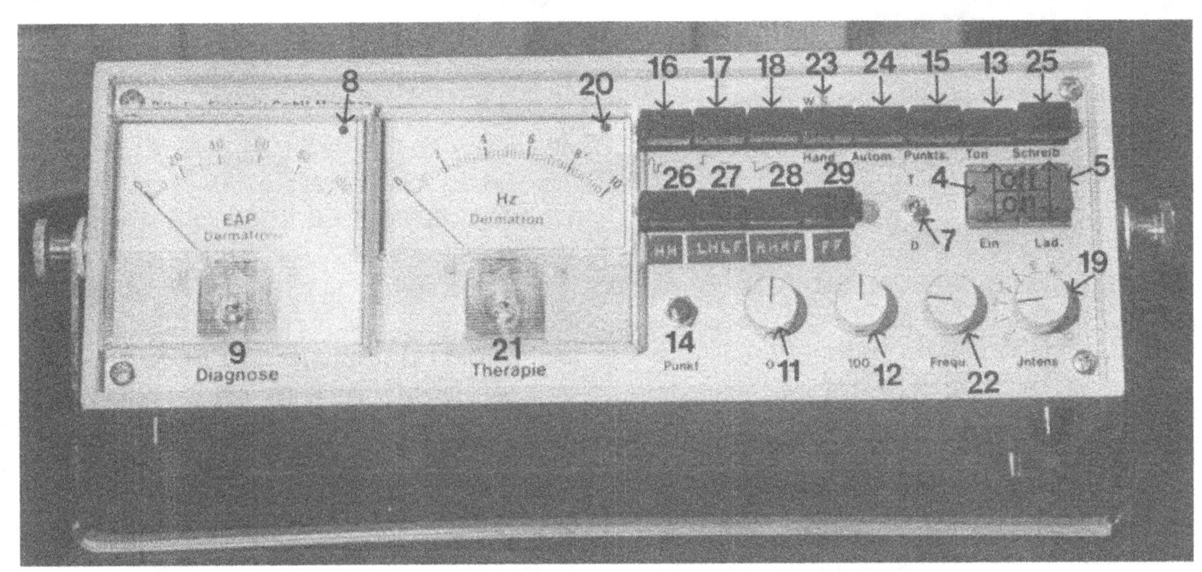

#8 RED LIGHT INDICATOR
#9 DIAGNOSIS OHMMETER
#20 RED LIGHT INDICATOR
#21 THERAPY OHMMETER
#14 PUNKT SKIN ACTIVATOR
#11 CALIBRATION KNOBS —ZERO
#12 CALIBRATION KNOBS —100
#22 REGULATOR —FOR FREQUENCY
#19 INTENSITY REGULATOR
#4 A/C MAIN SWITCH (GREEN)
#5 D/C CHARGE SWITCH (RED)
#7 TUMBLER SWITCH

#26 QUADRANT SELECTOR, I BUTTON
#27 QUADRANT SELECTOR, II BUTTON
#28 QUADRANT SELECTOR, III BUTTON
#29 QUADRANT SELECTOR, IV BUTTON
#16 THERAPY BUTTON (LASTING ENERGY)
#17 THERAPY BUTTON (SEDATION)
#18 THERAPY BUTTON (QUICK ENERGY)
#23 MANUAL BUTTON (WAVE SWING)
#24 AUTONOMIC BUTTON
#15 PUNKT BUTTON
#13 TON BUTTON
#25 PERIPHERAL EQUIPMENT BUTTON

PARTICULARS OF THE DERMATRON

TOP ROW BUTTONS

FIRST BUTTON — ENERGY. *Illustration 16 shows the first button which builds up energy slowly. It is good tor a long-lasting energy build up. The diagram underneath the button shows as low energy going up.*

1. To energize the patient, have the patient hold the BRASS ELECTRODES with the RED and BLACK PLUGS.

2. The feet are on the BRASS PLATES —YELLOW and GREEN PLUGS.

3. The POSITIVE POLES are on the right side — RED PLUG for the HAND ELECTRODE, GREEN PLUG for the FOOT PLATE.

4. The NEGATIVE POLES are on the left side — BLACK PLUG for the HAND ELECTRODE, YELLOW PLUG for the FOOT PLATE.

5. The frequency is **10 HZ** — illustration #22.

6. The intensity is set at **10** or as much as the patient can tolerate — illustration #19.

7. The tumbler switch is depressed to DIAGNOSIS — illustration #7.

8. The DIAGNOSIS OHMMETER should read **82** for all quadrants that are normal or free of pathological irritations — illustration #9.

9. The INDICATOR LIGHT should show RED when reading the DIAGNOSIS OHMMETER. This shows that it is operating in diagnosis rather than therapy— illustration #8.

SECOND ROW BUTTONS

1. I BUTTON indicates hand to hand which refers to the head, to the shoulder and trunk readings on both sides of the body.

2. II BUTTON indicates the left hand, left foot. This refers to the left side of the body.

3. III BUTTON indicates the right hand, right foot. This refers to the right side of the body.

4. IV BUTTON indicates the lower part of the body from the lower trunk to the lower extremities on both sides.

When one BUTTON is depressed, it will indicate

the status of that quadrant whether there is degeneration or inflammation. Normal readings are **82.** Below that is the degeneration of low energy. Above **82** is high energy and inflammation. If there is a difference in the quadrant reading of 10 or more, serious pathological problems could result. These values should be recorded on the EAV DENTAL CHART, third page.

The WAVESWING or MANUAL BUTTON, illustration #23, when out will produce a waveswing movement on the THERAPY OHMMETER, illustration #21, from **.8** to **10 HZ.** This low frequency current pulse generation can be continuously adjusted in frequency automatically from **.8** to **10 HZ** by an electronic circuit in the DERMATRON. By depressing the BUTTON, this low frequency current can be adjusted manually. Manual control, providing one knows the frequency works faster.

The general rule of thumb when using MANUAL CONTROL is that **.8 HZ** to **3.8 HZ** are for lymph and blood; **3.9 HZ** to **7** are for autonomic and peripheral nervous systems; and **7.1** to **10 HZ** are for organs and muscles.

In most cases, the WAVESWING BUTTON is out during therapy. Experience has shown that the therapeutic effect can be initiated more rapidly during treatment by varying the frequency from **.8 HZ** to **10 HZ,** from one current pulse to another, instead of using a fixed current.

During therapy, the WAVESWING will move from **.8 HZ** to **10 HZ** and then recycle itself again.

The AUTONOMIC BUTTON when depressed, illustration #24, can be used if the patient is left by himself. This will regulate the DIAGNOSIS METER alternately with the THERAPY METER every few seconds. This enables the patient or assistant to read the values on the diagnosis meter between therapy.

If the BUTTON is out, the operator must then manually move the TUMBLER SWITCH up for treatment and down for diagnosis, illustration #7.

The RED LIGHT INDICATOR will blink intermittently on diagnosis if used on therapy, illustrations #8, #20. This indicates to the operator which meter is being used. The TUMBLER SWITCH #7 will flash the THERAPY METER #21, the depressed level will light up the diagnosis meter #8. The frequency of the flashing light will be determined by the frequency applied. The higher the frequency the more rapid the flashing. For example, the flashing light blinks more rapidly at **10 HZ** than at **3 HZ.**

When the intensity is increased in the case of tonification, a pause must be provided after each alternating current pulse to prevent an overload. The patient must always be in a position to throw off the ELECTRODES if the current intensity becomes unpleasant. This insures that there will not be any prolonged type of contractions. The PUNKTS BUTTON, illustration #15, is used for the VARIPONT DIAGNOSTIC ELECTRODE. This is useful for the beginner and for verifying points that the operator is not familiar with. Do not depress this BUTTON when you are using the regular RED ELECTRODE because your DERMATRON will not work. This is only used for the VARIPONT ELECTRODE.

The TON BUTTON, illustration #13, is used as a sound finder. When applying the RED POSITIVE ELECTRODE to the acupuncture point, there will be a sound. As the operator applies more pressure to the point, the sound will increase in pitch. When the maximum intensity is reached (correct reading at this point), there will be a change in pitch or a "wobbling" sound which indicates to the operator that this is the reading at its maximum point. Increasing the pressure on the point serves no purpose other than to hurt the patient and overstimulate the point measured. This sound should be used to determine how much pressure is needed to find the maximum measurement value.

BUTTON #17 should be left out when energizing the patient. The last BUTTON on the top row is used for PERIPHERAL EQUIPMENT such as an AUXILLIARY METER. This is used for teaching purposes so all the students can see the METER. The **ZERO** FIGURE #11 and **100** FIGURE #12 CALIBRATION KNOBS should be balanced to **0** and **100.** Have the patient hold one BRASS ELECTRODE with the BLACK PLUG and the other BRASS ELECTRODE without any PLUG. The RED STYLUS ELECTRODE touches the interior portion of the BRASS ELECTRODE. If the reading is not **100,** the KNOB is adjusted to **100.** When the RED STYLUS is not touching the attached BATON, the reading on the DIAGNOSTIC METER should read ZERO. If not, adjust accordingly. If the METER cannot be adjusted to **100** when two HAND ELECTRODES are touched, then your battery is low. Also depress the SECOND ROW OF

BUTTONS first and SECOND BUTTONS to see if the METER hits **100.** If it doesn't, the BATTERY is low and must be recharged.

You are now ready to tonify the patient using the THIRD BUTTON, III TOP ROW BUTTONS. How long you energize the patient depends on how long it takes to bring his energy to **82.** If the patient is very low in energy, you may have to do several treatments to normalize him. Here the energy will fluctuate from a high to a low and back since it is being stabilized in the body. The energy is being moved from organs to secondary vessels and back to organs through the meridian circuits. Your readings on the SECOND ROW i, II, III, and **IV,** will determine whether you need to energize or sedate the patient. If the patient is low in energy, below **82,** then use the FIRST TOP ROW BUTTON. If the patient is in excess of **82,** use the SECOND BUTTON, sedation; and reduce it to **82.** When the patient is extremely low, **60** and below, use the THIRD BUTTON #18. This is true in cancer patients. For the FIRST and THIRD TOP ROW BUTTONS, use the same adjustment as described above. Sometimes you may want to depress both ONE and THREE TOP ROW BUTTONS together to stabilize and raise the energy faster. The THIRD TOP ROW BUTTON is used to bring the patient's energy up more rapidly but will not produce much stability as when using BUTTON ONE.

When the diagnostic procedure is completed, the patient must have values of **82** in order to have a consistent reading. In this instance, the hand-hand, illustration #26, is all that is needed to bring the energy up to **82.**

When healing therapy is used for the whole body, then completely balance the tonification and sedation of all quadrants, illustrations #26, #27, #28, and #29. This is especially advantageous in post surgery cases.

SECOND BUTTON — Sedation, illustration #17.

Sedation is used when the energy is too high and must be lowered. A majority of patients need to have their acupuncture points, and not quadrants, reduced. Lowering them to **50** value is 80 to 90 per cent of the problem. Don't sedate after 11:00 p.m. as the patient is in vagotonia, exhausted, and ready to go to sleep.

The setting — The frequency is usually on waveswing to **8 HZ.** The intensity is set from **.8** to **2.**

When treating a patient, it is ideal to treat his terminal measurement points on the hands and feet to **50.** This normalization will help preserve his energy as well as help the body rid itself of harmful diseases.

Press the BUTTON on the RED ELECTRODE until the NEEDLE on the DIAGNOSTIC METER drops down to ZERO. Release it and press again. Repeat this until the value drops to **50.**

Energizing the Acupuncture Points — The Build-up

When the patient has values on the acupuncture point below **50,** then tonify the points to **50.** These patients are in a degenerative stage. The settings are:

1. The intensity is usually set at **3** or more depending on the patient's pain tolerance. If it is uncomfortable for the patient, reduce the intensity.

2. When the patient first feels pain after the measurement exceeds **50,** stop immediately at this point. The patient should indicate when he first feels a tingling sensation so the therapist can stop increasing the intensity. If this is not done, there will be pain on the next step. In this way, the body protects itself against an overdose.

Techniques in Finding the Points

Most of the measurement points are located in the hands and feet in the proximal or distal head of the joints. The following has proven to be less painful than that found in Voll's book.

1. With the BRASS POINTS, the CROSS SLIT, illustration #120, is used. Refer to the illustration on all points. This SLIT holds the water.

2. Slide the HEAD OF THE POINT down the bone and tip the POINT FINDER up and into the concavity of the head of the joint.

3. Press in slightly and guide it with your left thumb.

4. Be sure that your left hand doesn't touch the patient, otherwise you may get a reading from your body.

5. Press down until you hear the pitch in the tone change has a wobbling sound.

6. You now can record the reading, and there is no need to press any harder.

PATIENT MANAGEMENT IN EAV

TREATMENT CONSENT FORM

The Consent Form Accomplishes Two Purposes:

1. The patient formally gives the doctor permission to use the EAV principle and other holistic practices. Since this instrument and discipline have not been accepted by the American Medical Association, it is necessary to inform the patient in writing that this is a research technique. When the patient consents to this in writing, legal problems can be avoided.

2. The patient accepts the responsibility of being treated by other than an orthodox method. The patient becomes part of the healing process, for the body cures itself, not the doctor. When the patient helps take care of his own body, the body's defensive mechanism is better able to repel diseases. This confirms the confidence shown by the patient in the doctor and contributes to the rapport. The patient soon becomes aware of progress and what is happening to his body through education and with professional guidance. The OHMMETER soon becomes very familiar to him. He participates and learns through experience how to take care of his body. The patient is then brought to good health throughout treatment. This builds up morale and motivation for him to continue this total health concept in the future. Costly medical and dental expenses can be drastically reduced. This is practicing preventative therapy.

3. The following is a sample copy of a Treatment Consent Form.

Acupuncture Form:

If one is to treat the body holistically, one must keep good records of the patient to monitor his progress. The following has been prepared specifically for this technique:

NOTES

Treatment Consent Form

The following is a sample of a Treatment Consent Form. It is advisable for you to have your attorney write one for you.

TREATMENT CONSENT FORM

Holistic natural healing using supplements such as vitamins, minerals, enzymes, glandular extracts and homeopathic remedies is becoming very popular in the treatment and prevention of oral dysfunctions, oral diseases as well as systemic imbalances.

In establishing a nutritional, structural and oral diagnosis, it is necessary to use various physical and technical diagnostic methods. Some of the methods have been established and accepted as standard office procedures. In order to continue to provide you with modern examination techniques and treatment procedures, research is required. Some of the testings used are still considered research. You will be informed of this if you require such testing for me to establish a diagnosis and treatment. It is also recommended that further x-ray and other standard laboratory tests from your physician be taken as a follow-up to our diagnosis.

If you decide not to take the x-rays and standard laboratory tests, then you will assume sole responsibility for this action.

This consent form will be placed in your chart for a permanent record. I have read, understand and accept the above information.

Patient's Signature Date

NOTES

NOTES

EAV Diagnosis and Treatment Chart

PAGE ONE Fig. 608

The tooth diagram is charted as a record for dental-related diseases. Two American nomenclatures are illustrated, the 1-32 and the 1-8. Five jaw sections are also illustrated.

Record the dates, any observations, and any dental irregularities under "comments."

PAGE TWO Fig. 609

A. Body energy — The quadrants signify the energy of **HH** — head and upper trunk; **LHLF** — left side of the body; **RHRF**— right side of the body; **FF** — lower trunk and extremities.

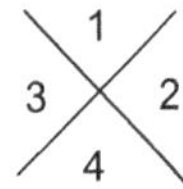

B. Record the values of each quadrant. The ideal value is **82.** Above **82** is inflammation, below **82** is degeneration.

C. The supplement explains all acupuncture points.

D. The maximum reading is recorded on the top half of the block. If there is an indicator drop, the lower half of the block denotes the lowest value of the INDICATOR DROP. If the maximum reading has no INDICATOR DROP, write the value on the top part of the block leaving the bottom of the block blank.

E. Remedy and dosages should be recorded as the medicine or natural supplement used with the dilution, capsule or tablets used. E.g., lungs using pertussin-3X or Real 15 tablets-(5). If more than one remedy is used, circle the appropriate blocks involved. Also circle the involved acupuncture point or points.

F. Indicate by an ARROW in the column whether the dosages should be GOING UP or DOWN.

G. Use different colors for each appointment for easy reading.

H. The second to fifth columns, which represent appointments, use the same procedures as the first. The sixth visit is written in the record section in this order:

1. Acupuncture points.
2. Right or left values with an indicator drop or a value that is stable.
3. Remedy and dosage.
4. Arrow either up or down for dosage pattern.

PAGE THREE

Starts the feet points.

PAGE FOUR

A. This page uses the same concept as page one and two.

B. The total column represents the number of indicator drops or inflammation collectivity.

C. The humoral, allergic and neural are the total number of each testing point of the hands and the feet. The humoral is the fluid balance of the body and usually is indicative of the kidney condition. The neural represents the nerve degeneration point while the allergy is related to its own meridian.

PAGE FIVE Fig 610

This page is to record the date and procedures of what has been done on each appointment. There is no need to record the remedy and dosage here except when exceeding the fifth visit.

PAGE SIX Fig 611

A. The ear illustration is used to record AURICULO-THERAPY.

B. The POSTURAL ANALYSIS is used to record any structural and muscular dysfunction. These can be illustrated by arrows in the direction of the pain and dysfunction. The date and particulars are written under comments.

C. The DERMATOMES are used to record scars and vertebrae deformities.

D. The MEDICAL-DENTAL HISTORIES are analyzed with the POSTURAL ANALYSIS and DERMATOMES and correlated to the particular tooth and its related organs and tissue systems. Circle each abnormality. The final record will show a pattern of the patient's total health. The next step is to find the cause of these symptoms and to follow the patient's progress with this chart.

NOTES

Fig. 608 — **EAV Diagnosis and Treatment Chart — Page 1**

REVISED E A V DIAGNOSIS & TREATMENT CHART

COMMENTS

PATIENT NAME: ______________________ DATE: ____________ No. _____

DENTAL EXAMINATION: ***OUTLINE DYSFUNCTIONS***

The energetic relations of teeth (or odontons) with respect to organs and tissue systems

	8 (1)	7, 6 (2, 3)	5, 4 (4, 5)	3 (6)	2, 1 (7, 8)	1, 2 (9, 10)	3 (11)	4, 5 (12, 13)	6, 7 (14, 15)	8 (16)
Endocrine glands	Anterior pituitary lobe	Para-thyroid / Thyroid	Thymus / Posterior pituitary lobe	Inter-mediate pituitary lobe	Pineal gland	Pineal gland	Posterior pituitary lobe	Inter-mediate pituitary lobe / Thymus	Thyroid / Para-thyroid	Anterior pituitary lobe
Sense organs	Internal ear Tongue	Tongue	Nose	Eye posterior portion	Nose	Nose	Eye posterior portion	Nose	Tongue	Internal ear Tongue
Paranasal sinuses	Cavernous Sinus	Maxillary sinus	Ethmoid cells	Sphenoidal sinus	Sphenoidal sinus / Frontal sinus	Sphenoidal sinus / Frontal sinus	Sphenoidal sinus	Ethmoid cells	Maxillary sinus	Cavernous Sinus
Joints	Shoulder ul s Elbow ul s Hand, ulnar side	Jaw	Shoulder ra s Elbow ra s Hand radial side	Posterior knee / Hip	Posterior knee / sacro coccygeal joint	Posterior knee / sacro coccygeal joint	Posterior knee / Hip	Shoulder ra s Elbow ra s Hand radial side	Jaw	Shoulder ul s Elbow ul s Hand, ulnar side
	Foot, plantar side Toes	Anterior hip Anterior knee Medical ankle joint	Foot Big toe	Ankle joint	Ankle joint	Ankle joint	Ankle joint	Foot Big toe	Anterior hip Anterior knee Medical ankle joint	Foot, plantar side Toes
	Sacro iliac joint			lateral	posterior	posterior	lateral			Sacro iliac joint
Segments of the spinal marrow and Dermatomes	SC2 SC1 STh1 SC8 STh 7 STh6 STh5 SS2 SS1	SC2 SC1 STh12 STh11 SL1	SC2 SC1 SC5 SC6 SC7 STh2 STh3 STh4 SL4 SL5	SC2 SC1 STh8 STh9 STh 10	SC2 SC1 SL3 SL 2 SCo SS5 SS4 SS3	SC1 SC2 SL2 SL3 SS3 SS4 SS5 SCo	SC1 SC2 STh 8 STh 9 STh 10	SC1 SC2 SC5 SC6 SC7 STh2 STh3 STh4 SL4 SL5	SC1 SC2 STh11 STh12 SL1	SC1 SC2 SC8 STh1 STh5 STh6 STh7 SS1 SS2
Vertebrae	C2 C1 TH1 C7 Th7 Th6 Th5 S2 S1	C2 C1 TH12 Th11 L1	C2 C1 C7 C6 C5 Th 4 Th3 Th2 L5 L4	C2 C1 TH8 Th9 Th10	C2 C1 L3 L2 Co S5 S4 S3	C1 C2 L2 L3 S3 S4 S5 Co	C1 C2 TH8 Th9 Th10	C1 C2 C5 C6 C7 Th3 Th4 L4 L5	C1 C2 TH11 TH12 L1	C1 C2 C7 TH1 Th5 Th6 Th7 S1 S2
Organs Yang	Heart right side	Pancreas	Lung right side	Liver right side	Kidney right side	Kidney left side	Liver left side	Lung left side	Spleen	Heart left side
Organs Yin	Duodenum right side Terminal ileum	Oesophagus Stomach, right side	Large intestine right side	Gall-bladder Biliary ducts right side	Urinary bladder. right side Genito-urinary area Rectum Anal Canal	Urinary bladder. left side Genito-urinary area Rectum Anal Canal	Biliary ducts left side	Large intestine left side	Oesophagus Stomach, left side	Duodenum left side jejunum ileum
Cranial Nerves	8, 9, 12	9, 12	1, 5	2	1, 5	1, 5	2	1, 5	9, 12	8, 9, 12
Tissue systems	Central nervous system Limbic system									Central nervous system Limbic system
Other systems	Depression Tinnitus	Mammary gland right side							Mammary gland left side	Depression Tinnitus
Jaw sections	HE.,CS.,SI	ST. IV PA.	LI. III LU.	Liv. GB	BL. I KI.	KI. I BL.	Liv. GB	LU. III LI.	SP. IV ST.	HE., CS., SI.
American nomenclature	1	2 / 3	4 / 5	6	7 / 8	9 / 10	11	12 / 13	14 / 15	16
Tonsils	Lingual	Laryngeal	Tubal	Pal.	Pharyngeal	Pharyngeal	Pal.	Tubal	Laryngeal	Lingual
Teeth diegram	right									left
Tooth number	8 +	7 + / 6 +	5 + / 4 +	3 +	2 + / 1 +	+ 1 / + 2	+ 3	+ 4 / + 5	+ 6 / + 7	+ 8
Tooth number	8 -	7 - / 6 -	5 - / 4 -	3 -	2 - / 1 -	- 1 / - 2	- 3	- 4 / - 5	- 6 / - 7	- 8
Teeth diegram	right (retro-molar)									(retro-molar) left
Tonsils	Lingual	Tubal	Laryngeal	Pal.	Pharyngeal	Pharyngeal	Pal.	Laryngeal	Tubal	Lingual
American nomenclature	Kidney Adrenal	31 / 30	29 / 28	27	26 / 25	24 / 23	22	21 / 20	19 / 18	Kidney Adrenal
Jaw sections	HE.,CS.,SI	LI. IV LU.	ST. III PA.	Liv. GB	BL. I KI.	KI. I BL.	Liv. GB	SP. III ST.	LU. IV LI.	HE., CS., SI.
Other systems	Energy exchange		Mammary gland right side					Mammary gland left side		Energy exchange
Tissue systems	Peripheral nerves	Arteries / Veins	Lymph vessels	3, 4, 5,	Sacral Pelvic Splanchici	Sacral Pelvic Splanchic	3, 4, 5,	Lymph vessels	Veins / Arteries	Peripheral nerves
Cranial Nerves	5, 7, 12	5, 10, 11	5, 10, 12	6, 11			6, 11	5, 10, 12	5, 10, 11	5, 7, 12
Organs Yin	Terminal ileum / Ileo cecal area	Large intestine right side / Ileo cecal area	Oesophagus Stomach, right side pylorus Pyloric antrum	Gall bladder Biliary ducts right side	Rectum Anal canal Urinary bladder right side genito Urinary area	Rectum Anal canal Urinary bladder left side genito Urinary area	Billary ducts left side	Oesophagus Stomach, left side	Large intestine left side	Jejunum Ileum. left side
Organs Yang	Heart right side	Lung right side	Pancreas	Liver right side	Kidney right side	Kidney left side	Liver left side	Spleen	Lung left side	Heart left side
Vertebral	C2 C1 Th1 C7 Th7 Th6 Th5 S2 S1	C2 C1 C7 C6 C5 Th4 Th3 L5 L4	C2 C1 Th 12 Th11 L1	C2 C1 TH8 Th9 Th10	C2 C1 L3 L2 S5 S4 S3 Co	C1 C2 L2 L3 S3 S4 S5 Co	C1 C2 TH8 Th9 Th10	C1 C2 Th11 Th12 L1	C1 C2 C5 C6 C7 Th3 Th4 L4 L5	C1 C2 C7 Th1 Th5 Th6 Th7 S1 S2
Segments of the spinal marrow and Dermatomes	SC2 SC1 STh1 SC8 STh 7 STh6 STh5 SS2 SS1	SC2 SC1 Sc7 SC6 SC5 STh4 STh3 STh5 SL5 SL4	SC2 SC1 STh12 STh11 SL1	SC2 SC1 STh8 STh9 STh 10	SC2 SC1 SL3 SL 2 SCo SS5 SS4	SC1 SC2 SL2 SL3 SS4 SS5 SCo	SC1 SC2 STh 8 STh 9 STh 10	SC1 SC2 STh11 STh12 SL1	SC1 SC2 SC5 SC6 SC7 STh2 STh3 STh4 SL4 SL5	SC1 SC2 SC8 STh1 STh5 STh6 STh7 SS1 SS2
Joints	Shoulder Elbow right side	Shoulder Elbow right side	Anterior hip Anterior knee	Posterior knee	Posterior knee	Posterior knee	Posterior knee	Anterior hip Anterior knee	Shoulder Elbow left side	Shoulder Elbow left side
	Hand, ulnar side Foot plantar side Toes	Hand radial side Foot Big toe	Medial ankle joint	Hip	Sacro-coccygeal joint	Sacro-coccygeal joint	Hip	Medial ankle joint	Hand radial side Foot Big toe	Hand, ulnar side Foot plantar side Toes
	Sacro-iliac joint		Jaw	Ankle joint lateral	Ankle joint posterior	Ankle joint posterior	Ankle joint lateral	Jaw		Sacro-iliac joint
Paranasal sinuses		Ethmoid cells	Maxillary sinus	Sphenoidal sinus	Frontal sinus / Sphenoidal sinus	Frontal sinus / Sphenoidal sinus	Sphenoidal sinus	Maxillary sinus	Ethmoid cells	
Sense organs	Middle external ear Tongue	Nose	Tongue	Eye anterior portion	Nose	Nose	Eye anterior portion	Tongue	Nose	Middle external ear Tongue
Endocrine glands			Gonad	Gonad	Adrenal gland	Adrenal gland	Gonad			

Original E.A.V DIAGNOSIS and TREATMENT CHART by Reinhold Voll. M.D

Interrelations of Odontons and Tonsils to Organs. Field of Disturbances and Tissue System. Published by M. L. Publishers. D311 Uelzen, West Germany

Fig. 609 — **EAV Diagnosis and Treatment Chart — Pages 2, 3, 4**

Body Energy - Quadrant:

1. H.H. = Hand - Hand
2. LHLF = Left hand, Left foot
3. RHRF = Right hand, Right foot
4. FF = Foot, Foot

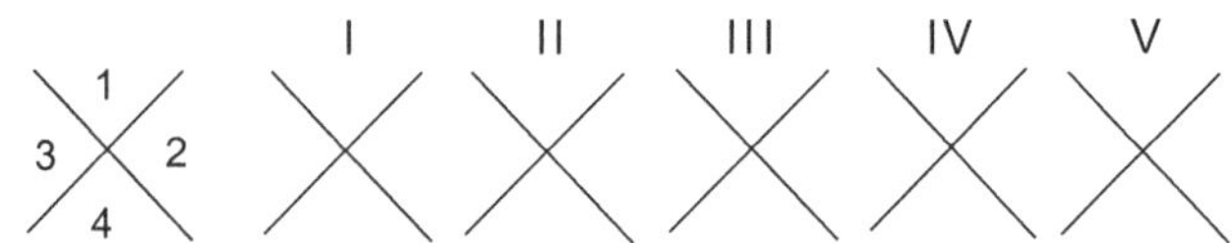

HANDS	R	L	Remedy Dosage	M.P.	R	L	Remedy Dosage	M.P.	R	L	Remedy Dosage	M.P.	R	L	Remedy Dosage	M.P.	R	L	
LY - 1																			
LY - 1-1																			
Ton. Ring																			
LY - 2																			
2a Eye																			
LY - 3																			
LU- 11																			
LU -10d																			
CMP																			
LU - 10b																			
LU - 10a																			
LU - 10																			
LI - 1																			
CMP																			
Peritoneum																			
LI - 2																			
LI - 3																			
LI - 4																			
Lt - 4a																			
Ne - 1																			
Auto.																			
CMP																			
Men.																			
Ne - 2																			
Ne - 3																			
Ne - 3a																			
Ne - 4																			
Ci - 9																			
CMP																			
Ci - 8																			
Ci - 7																			

	R	L	Remedy Dosage	M.P.	R	L	Remedy Dosage	M.P.	R	L	Remedy Dosage	M.P.	R	L	Remedy Dosage	M.P.	R	L	Remedy Dosage
All - 1																			
CMP																			
Va. SCl.																			
All - 2																			
All - 3																			
Or - 1																			
CMP																			
Peritoneum																			
Pleura.																			
Or - 2																			
Or - 3																			
TW- 1																			
CMP																			
Pa																			
Ma. Gl.																			
TW - 2																			
TW - 3																			
He -9																			
CMP																			
He -8a																			
He -8																			
He- 7																			
He -6																			
S.I. -1																			
CMP																			
S.I. - 2																			
S.I. - 3																			

TOTAL

FEET

	R	L	Remedy Dosage	M.P.	R	L	Remedy Dosage	M.P.	R	L	Remedy Dosage	M.P.	R	L	Remedy Dosage	M.P.	R	L	Remedy Dosage
Pa.- 1, Sp-1																			
CMP																			
Pa. -2, Sp - 2																			
Pa. -3, Sp- 3																			
Pa. -4																			
Liv.- 1																			
CMP																			
Liv. - 2																			
Liv. - 3																			

	R	L	Remedy Dosage	M.P.	R	L	Remedy Dosage	M.P.	R	L	Remedy Dosage	M.P.	R	L	Remedy Dosage	M.P.	R	L	Remedy Dosage
Jo. - 1																			
CMP																			
Syn. Me.																			
Jo. - 2																			
Jo. - 3																			
St. 45																			
Coe Pl.																			
CMP																			
Fib. - 1																			
CMP																			
Fib. - 2																			
Fib. - 3																			
SK- 1																			
Scar																			
SK - 2																			
SK - 3																			
Fat. - 1																			
CMP																			
Fat. - 2																			
Fat. - 3																			
GBL 44																			
CMP																			
GBL - .																			
Ki - 1																			
Ki - 1-1																			
CMP																			
Ki - 1b																			
UB - 67																			
CMP																			
UB - 65																			
TOTAL																			

Humoral__________ Allergic__________ Neural__________

Hypothalamus__________ , __________

Fig. 610 — **EAV Diagnosis and Treatment Chart — Page 5**

RECORDS

DATE: ______________________

Fig. 611 — **EAV Diagnosis and Treatment Chart — Page 6**

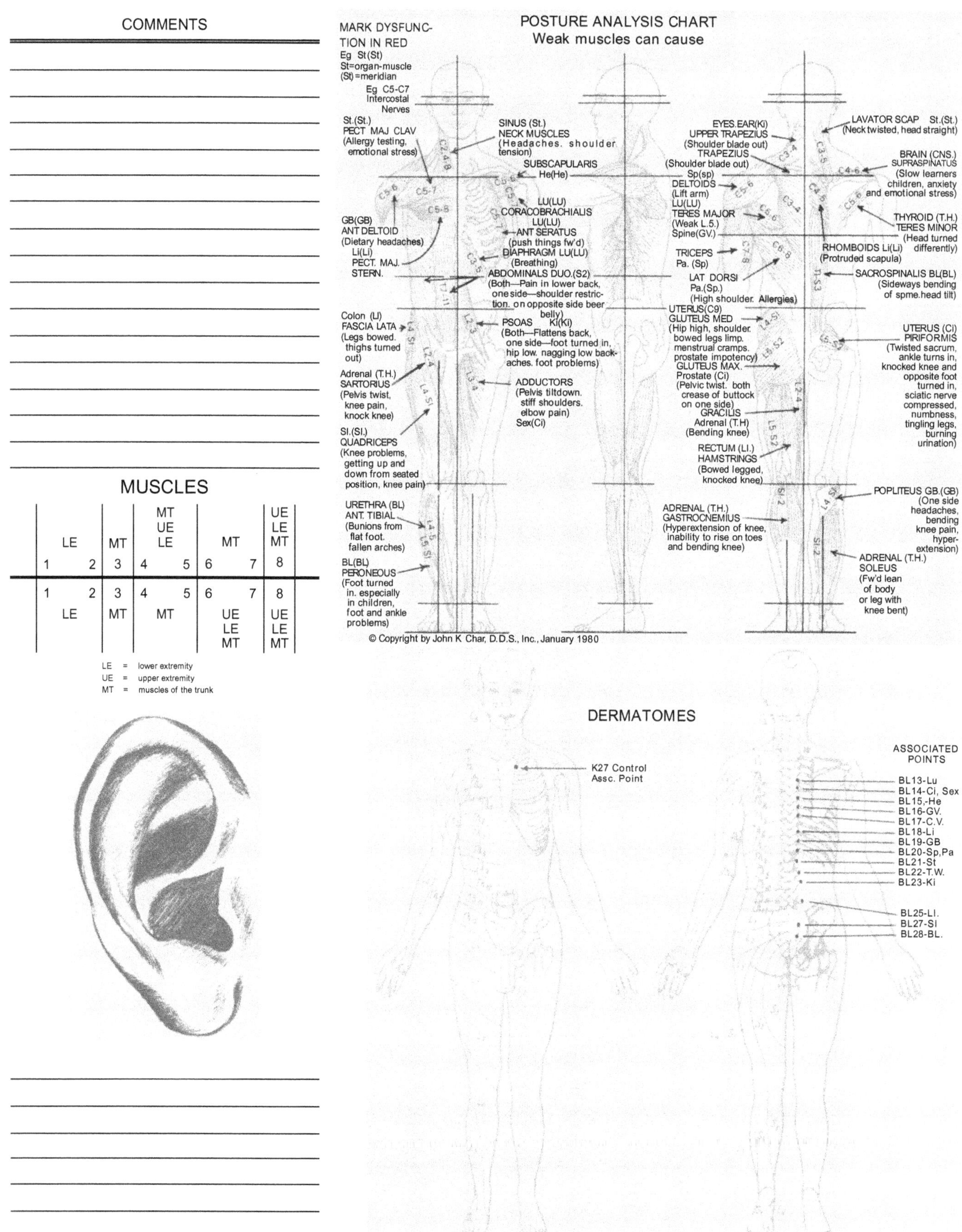

COMMENTS
MUSCLES
MT UE LE
UE LE MT
LE
MT
MT
1 2 3 4 5 6 7 8
1 2 3 4 5 6 7 8
LE
MT
MT
UE LE MT
UE LE MT
LE = lower extremity
UE = upper extremity
MT = muscles of the trunk
POSTURE ANALYSIS CHART
Weak muscles can cause
MARK DYSFUNCTION IN RED
Eg St(St)
St=organ-muscle
(St)=meridian
Eg C5-C7 Intercostal Nerves
St.(St.) PECT MAJ CLAV (Allergy testing, emotional stress)
GB(GB) ANT DELTOID (Dietary headaches)
Li(Li) PECT. MAJ. STERN.
Colon (LI) FASCIA LATA (Legs bowed. thighs turned out)
Adrenal (T.H.) SARTORIUS (Pelvis twist, knee pain, knock knee)
SI.(SI.) QUADRICEPS (Knee problems, getting up and down from seated position, knee pain)
URETHRA (BL) ANT. TIBIAL (Bunions from flat foot. fallen arches)
BL(BL) PERONEOUS (Foot turned in. especially in children, foot and ankle problems)
SINUS (St.) NECK MUSCLES (Headaches. shoulder tension)
SUBSCAPULARIS He(He)
LU(LU) CORACOBRACHIALIS
LU(LU) ANT SERATUS (push things fw'd)
DIAPHRAGM LU(LU) (Breathing)
ABDOMINALS DUO.(S2) (Both—Pain in lower back, one side—shoulder restriction. on opposite side beer belly)
PSOAS Ki(Ki) (Both—Flattens back, one side—foot turned in, hip low. nagging low back-aches. foot problems)
ADDUCTORS (Pelvis tiltdown. stiff shoulders. elbow pain) Sex(Ci)
EYES.EAR(Ki) UPPER TRAPEZIUS (Shoulder blade out)
TRAPEZIUS (Shoulder blade out)
Sp(sp) DELTOIDS (Lift arm)
LU(LU) TERES MAJOR (Weak L.5.)
Spine(GV.)
TRICEPS Pa. (Sp)
LAT DORSI Pa.(Sp.) (High shoulder. Allergies)
UTERUS(C9) GLUTEUS MED (Hip high, shoulder. bowed legs limp. menstrual cramps. prostate impotency)
GLUTEUS MAX. Prostate (Ci) (Pelvic twist. both crease of buttock on one side)
GRACILIS Adrenal (T.H) (Bending knee)
RECTUM (LI.) HAMSTRINGS (Bowed legged, knocked knee)
ADRENAL (T.H.) GASTROCNEMIUS (Hyperextension of knee, inability to rise on toes and bending knee)
LAVATOR SCAP St.(St.) (Neck twisted, head straight)
BRAIN (CNS.) SUPRASPINATUS (Slow learners children, anxiety and emotional stress)
THYROID (T.H.) TERES MINOR (Head turned differently)
RHOMBOIDS Li(Li) (Protruded scapula)
SACROSPINALIS BL(BL) (Sideways bending of spme.head tilt)
UTERUS (Ci) PIRIFORMIS (Twisted sacrum, ankle turns in, knocked knee and opposite foot turned in, sciatic nerve compressed, numbness, tingling legs, burning urination)
POPLITEUS GB.(GB) (One side headaches, bending knee pain, hyper-extension)
ADRENAL (T.H.) SOLEUS (Fw'd lean of body or leg with knee bent)
© Copyright by John K Char, D.D.S., Inc., January 1980
DERMATOMES
K27 Control Assc. Point
ASSOCIATED POINTS
BL13-Lu
BL14-Ci, Sex
BL15,-He
BL16-GV.
BL17-C.V.
BL18-Li
BL19-GB
BL20-Sp,Pa
BL21-St
BL22-T.W.
BL23-Ki
BL25-LI.
BL27-SI
BL28-BL.
©Copyright by John K Char, D.D.S., Inc., January 1980

Control Measurement Points

There are 20 CONTROL MEASUREMENT POINTS located on the HANDS and FEET. TWO are found along the spine. TWELVE are on classical Chinese acupuncture meridians while EIGHT are Voll's measurements. The control points include those for the organs, circulation, endocrine, allergy, degenerative systems and the lymphatic vessels. All of them are located in the MIDDLE JOINTS of the FINGERS and TOES. By measuring these control points, you can quickly determine whether there is an acute or subacute inflammation, an organic degenerative event or focal disturbances taking place. This saves you valuable time. If the CONTROL MEASUREMENT POINT shows an INDICATOR DEFLECTION or a high degree of inflammation,then the related measurement on that meridian must be gauged.Thus, the maximum for the illness event can be found rapidly. It also pinpoints the patient's most immediate complaint through these indicative points and helps you arrive at an accurate diagnosis with the written medical history.

Most of these CONTROL POINTS can be palpated prior to the measurement of each point.

Other ACUPUNCTURE POINTS are located directly over certain bones. They are usually located above the bones at the transition from the shaft to the thickened initial and terminal portions. In other words, at bone angles that are easily felt. They can also be located above depressions and elevations on the bones, over interarticular spaces, above furrows in the joint cartilage, or above certain muscle locations. Acupuncture points are located above muscle margin angles or two or three muscle margins. These acupuncture points can also be felt above soft parts or above muscle margins.

Things to Consider before Measurement

☐ You must have the patient calibrated to **82** on the connected electrode to insure a consistent reading.

☐ The patient should be eating regularly since fasting weakens the patient. No sugar or irritants like coffee or alcohol should be taken a day before the measurement appointment. A person low in energy after fasting would not affect the reading as such. Rather, he is tender and the points are sore because the metabolism is shaky. When you add energy, the response is vehement but will not throw the readings off.

☐ Synthetics, like nylons, should not be worn as it can impede the energetic circulation because the constant rubbing of the material causes static and impedes the flow of energy to the meridians. Garters can also affect the meridian. The body's pH level can also affect the energy flow. Wigs may also impede the measurement value. Cotton, wool and silk are the best materials to wear. The patient should also wear loose-fitting clothing so it is easier to measure. Synthetic materials (nylon, plastics) may make the body hard to charge. This is because the material already has the charge on the surface. The superimposed charge by the measurement instrument does not make itself felt. Have the patient return the next day wearing cotton. Pink colored clothing should be avoided as it can reduce the body's energy.

☐ The patient should have a good night's sleep so he will be recharged.

☐ If there is cold and wet weather conditions, the recharging is difficult. According to classical acupuncture, you should not use acupuncture under certain weather conditions. When the weather is bad, the patient should test at 10:00 a.m. to 11:00 a.m. when all energy factors are highest. The season will give you different readings. There can be no polarization of the points through repeated testing. Barometric pressure, unless it supersedes a certain limit value, does not affect the readings, whereas electrical environment does. This refers to the lamps and mains of electric equipment. Electrical environment caused by atmospheric conditions such as lightning and electrical ions in the air can cause changes seen as measurements which can affect everybody and will give slight deviations either higher or lower. Full moon does not affect the readings.

☐ At night, the basic value goes down because of the vagotonia and there are fewer ID's than during the day. When children suddenly get tired at night, readings show **20** to **30;** they go from symphaticotonia to vagotonia (tiredness). Do not measure after 8:00 p.m. because the patient is in vagotonia.

☐ For those patients who have wet hands, have them wash their hands in cold water over the wrist and palms. The sweat causes a high concentration which impedes the measurement and shows high measurement values.

☐ Make sure there is no loose connection on the Dermatron. Make sure that the ELECTRODE POINTS of the STYLUS are not oxidized at the "screwed in" connection. If the values are higher than **82,** the patient is in a state of symphaticotonia which is normal. If the initial conductance measurement reading is below 82, check if the palms are wet enough. Use tap water on the ELECTRODES. This instrument is made to respond to tap water. If the indicator does not get as high or higher than **82,** that person may be suffering from a malignant process or did not sleep enough. It can be drug-caused too. Frequently, premalignancy is found when values taken hand to hand are low.

☐ You can use a WOODEN ROLLER on the soles of the feet for 10 to 20 minutes until the skin turns red. This energizes the feet. You have in effect stimulated the lymphatic and vascular system, and this will stimulate the healing process. You can perform procedures more rapidly and increase the energy. The patient should rest his feet on a WOODEN PODIUM with a cotton cloth placed over it.

☐ When a patient has a low reading, have the patient perform knee bends to bring the level up for a good reading.

☐ If the procedures are still not successful, apply ACID REMEDIES in potencies of **D3** intermuscularly. ACETIC ACID, PHOSPHORIC ACID, and CITRIC ACID increase internal metabolism. The energy increase is similar to a battery function. When the patient is at **50,** injecting intermuscularly will raise the values to about **75.** Have the patient return the next morning and energize a few days. The patient should be measurable.

☐ The doctor should wear cotton gloves or cover his hands with tissue paper if he has wet hands.

☐ If a low reading exists, check four quadrants for the body's energy. The BLACK BUTTONS are located on the second row labeled: **I-HH** (hand-hand which is the head and trunk quadrant).

II-LHLF (left hand-left foot which is the left part of the body).

III-RHRF (right hand-right foot which is the right half of the body).

IV-FF (foot-foot which is the quadrant from the hip to the foot).

By having the patient hold the BRASS ELECTRODES with RED and BLACK PLUGS and the GREEN and YELLOW PLUGS connected to the FOOT PLATES, you will be able to determine the energy measurement of each quadrant. If the reading is lower than **82** on any quadrant, the patient lacks sufficient energy in that area. Any reading in excess of **82** indicates an inflammation in that quadrant. Anything lower than **50** indicates degeneration in that quadrant. If the high reading and lowest reading deviate more than **10,** then something is wrong. For example:

We have degeneration on the left side of the body, BUTTON **II, 30** value. There is also inflammation on the upper portion of the body, **I** and **III,** values **88.** If you raise the low value **30** up to **82** then that quadrant pair will be energized. It is best to treat specific lymph points for inflammation. If this is not sufficient, then treat by the hand-hand electrode method.

You can sedate quadrant **I** and **III** and tonify **II:** sedation is accomplished by depressing the SECOND BUTTON on the upper row and BUTTONS

I, III on the second row. The adjustment is made on frequency **.8 to 10 HZ** and intensity **1-2.** The WAVESWING BUTTON can be depressed on the hand for a fixed frequency. For alternating frequencies, the WAVESWING BUTTON is elevated. The AUTOMATIC BUTTON METER reading is used as therapy and to diagnose. If automatic is not used, then the TREATMENT SWITCH is elevated. Each step needs to be separated if there is a need to tonify or sedate the quadrant involved. There are four quadrants: **HH, LHLF, RHRF,** and **FF.**

a. If these quadrants differ 10 schedulents, the person is in a state of energetic deficiency.

b. In order to establish proper punctual readings, you should recharge the person to the optimum intensity.

c. Time the frequency up to **10 HZ** or as high as the patient can tolerate. You use a high frequency rather than a lower frequency because the number of pulses per second carries out the recharging process.

d. One impulse per second takes longer than more frequent impulses.

e. This is accomplished by depressing the WAVESWING KEY.

f. Depress the 3RD KEY on the first row for the maximum energy.

g. This takes 10 minutes.

h. The therapeutic significance is effective.

i. You need to only charge the **HH** which takes care of the other quadrants.

j. The quadrants individually only check up on the respective locations of energetic insufficiencies in the body.

☐ The fluctuating values seen on the OHMMETER while energizing the patient is due to a circulation of stabilized energy which is recharging the superficial and deep reservoir supply of all individual organs. Through classical acupuncture, there are wonder vessels which are connecting vessels from meridian to meridian that follow certain pathways. These are also called secondary vessels. These secondary vessels have safeguards as to where this energy can be channeled into the deep areas or more superficial areas. When the OHM READING fluctuates **(68, 70, 72, 74, 72, 74, 76, 78, 74, 76, 80, etc.)** this does not mean energy is lost. The charges you add are led off to fill the energetic reservoir.

☐ By measuring, the patient tends to lose some energy. Charge the patient more than **82**. It is better to increase the energy in intervals in different quadrants of the body.

☐ Use the left OHMMETER in MICRO AMPS for diagnosis.

☐ It uses a direct current.

☐ When taking a reading on the **MP**, feed a certain current into the organ system, which travels along the meridian to get in contact with the organ tissue, and the response or interaction between the organ and the current is your final measurement reading.

☐ This results in various stages — inflammatory, normal and degenerative.

☐ As far as we know, the DERMATRON does not affect a pacemaker because the DERMATRON machine's current is low. However, be careful with this patient.

☐ The WAVE FORM is a given data in the machine and you can't change them. Only the frequency can be changed.

☐ There is no value too high for this instrument.

☐ The patient should not be grounded when you measure him. If he is, he will lose a lot of energy and will never get a proper reading.

☐ The patient should not be too close to the MAIN SWITCHBOX; he should be at least one meter and a half away (4 feet). The patient should not be right in front of the wall of the mains, which will affect your readings (either too high or too low).

☐ No bright lights should be on top of the patient's head, since that can influence the measurements.

☐ No x-ray machine or medical apparatus should be in the direct vicinity.

☐ No plugs should be under the examining table.

☐ The first thorough diagnosis and the follow-up diagnosis should be comparable rather than have too much of a difference.

☐ The mental functions (barring sleep) have no implications on the proper readings.

☐ By pressing too hard, you may overstimulate a point.

☐ Press on one location in order to establish a reading on the same acupuncture point and shift the electrode slightly. Then press the skin towards the location where you expect the acupuncture point to lie.

☐ You may shift the skin to the area where you expect the acupuncture point to lie.

☐ Different tissues make up the acupuncture points. The points are not situated on the outer skin nor are they on the periosteum.

☐ You will only throw the readings off when you have a serious illness.

☐ A person with high fever would not influence the reading other than these acupuncture points are high in the inflammatory stage in the organs affected.

☐ Being angry does not affect the readings.

☐ Energy will produce measurement values that are higher for energy involving the whole body. When the body is reactive or responsible to that, you will get high values because inflammation or irritation is bound to be present.

☐ Air ionization will have small effects which should be lightly considered.

☐ Although the position you measure is of little importance, the best measuring position is the sitting position.

☐ The new points found by Voll have a cyclic activity (such as the lymph point). They are associated with the organs and the lymph and are part of the organ to which they are attached. There is no maximum to the lymph cycle whereas in circulation, this depends on the heart and is limited to the heart.

☐ Metal jewelry on the patient interferes with the measurement process.

Testing the Dermatron for Charge

A. Hold two ELECTRODES together (short-circuit) to get a maximum reading of **100**. This shows that the ACCUMULATOR is charged.

B. Depress the first TWO KEYS in the second row. This will show **100** if the ACCUMULATOR is charged.

C. If every point shows a reading of **20** to **30**, be sure that your ACCUMULATOR is charged. This is usually possible unless something very severe interferes.

D. It is impossible to overcharge the machine.

E. It takes 10 hours to charge the DERMATRON.

F. The DERMATRON holds a charge for 2 days.

G. The **100** KNOB should be 1 to 3 o'clock position. If it reaches 3:00, the DERMATRON is almost empty and you must recharge it. Its normal position is 12 o'clock.

NOTES

HAND ELECTRO-ACUPUNCTURE POINTS ACCORDING TO VOLL

All acupuncture points found by Voll are done in anatomic plates to the bone and the points on the bone. There are many other points which are explained in Voll's books

Lymph Drainage

Voll's *Illustrated Volume II*, fig. 5, p. 19; fig. 6, p. 21.

1. MP-1 — Palatine Tonsil (may affect the liver).
2. MP-1 -1 — Ear (foci of the ear-tinnitus may affect the kidney and small intestine).
3. Tonsillar ring with 5 tonsils.
4. MP-1 a — Lat. lymphatic duct, tubal tonsil.
5. MP-2 — Dental (foci of upper and lower jaw).
6. MP-2a — Eye (eliminate toxins through organs first).
7. MP-3 — Nose, paranasal sinus.
8. *MP-4 — Lung — hiatus of lymph glands (children 7-9 years with constant cough without mucous).*
9. *MP-4a — Esophagus (one of the poorest organ to diagnose).*
10. *MP-4b — Larynx (hypolarynx).*
11. *MP-5 — Heart — may affect CI MP-7 — coronary vessels.*
12. *MP-6 — Lung, large intestine, circulation, endocrine. Lymph vessel of upper extremities.*
13. *MP-7 — Small intestine and duodenum.*
14. *MP-8 — Large intestine and rectum including chylous vessels.*
15. *MP-8a — Larynx.*
16. *MP-8b — Hypolarynx (lower part of larynx) measurement of 60-70 with chronic cough. (ID on MP-8a, 8b are signs of chronic laryngitis or chronic hyprocricord with little mucous).*
17. MP-9 — Endocrine gland.
18. MP-10 — Lymph nodes of abdomen, accompanying large blood vessels of the abdomen.
19. MP-11 — Situated on G.B. meridian. It possesses most secondary vessels (6). Three passes through the endocrine glands: parathyroid, thyroid, thymus. Three passes through the spleen: pancreas, liver, kidney.
20. MP-12 — Situated on L.I. meridian. Direct connection with medulla oblongata BL-10 and vertebral spine BL-11.
21. MP-13 — Situated on T.B. meridian. Organs of biliary functions, deep lying paranasal sinuses, ethmoid cells, sphenoidal sinus, sympathetic nerves, middle and internal ear (useful for drippy nose).
22. MP-14 — Situated on S.I. meridian. Maxillary sinus, genito-urinary organs, vertebral spine, frontal sinus, pineal gland, suprarenal gland (useful for roaming pain in body).

NOTES

Lymph Drainage

2. MP-1-1 — Ear (foci of the ear- tinnitus may affect the kidney and small intestine).

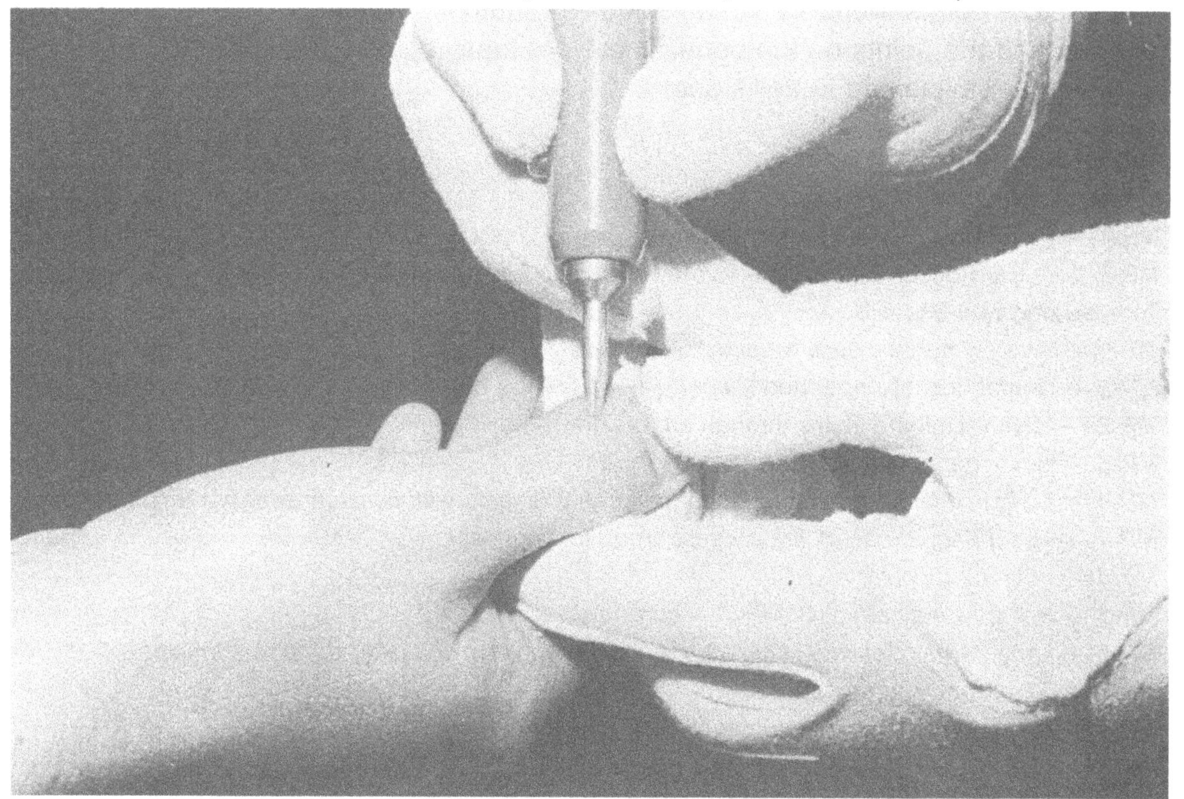

Lymph Drainage

3. Tonsillar ring with 5 tonsils.

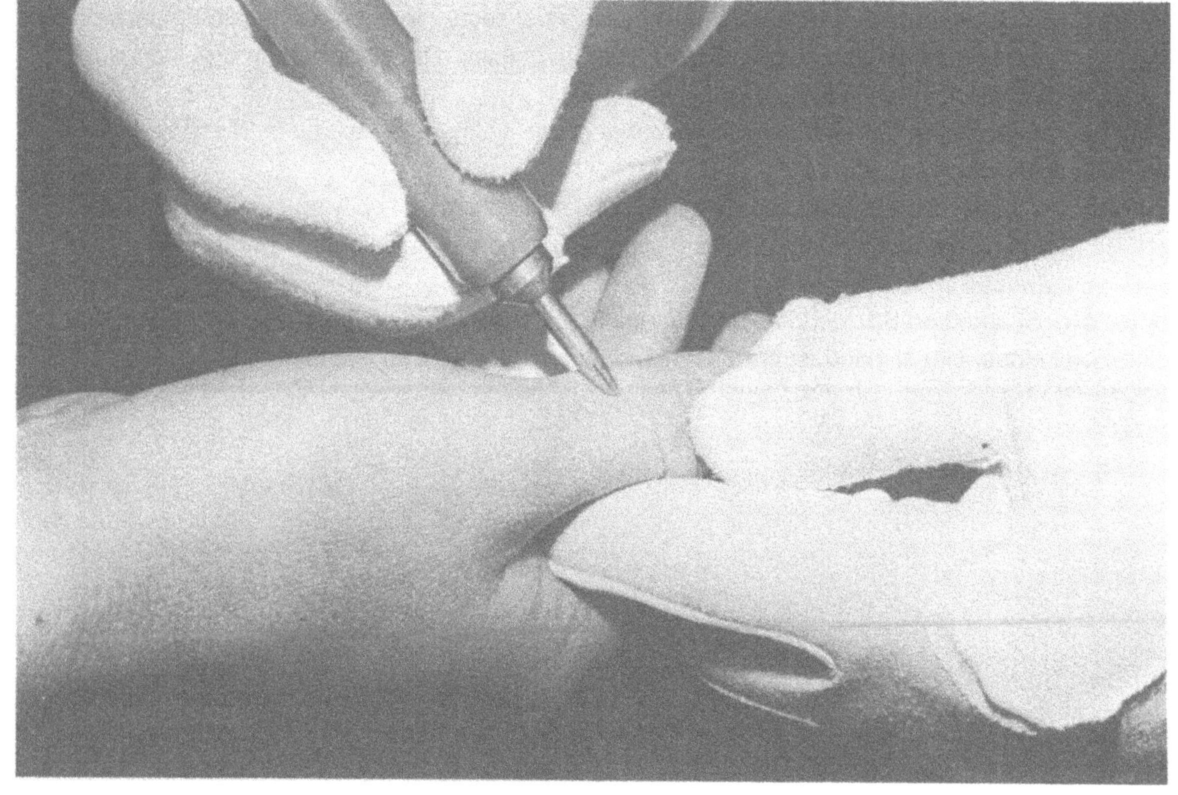

Lymph Drainage

5. MP-2 — Dental (foci of upper and lower jaw).

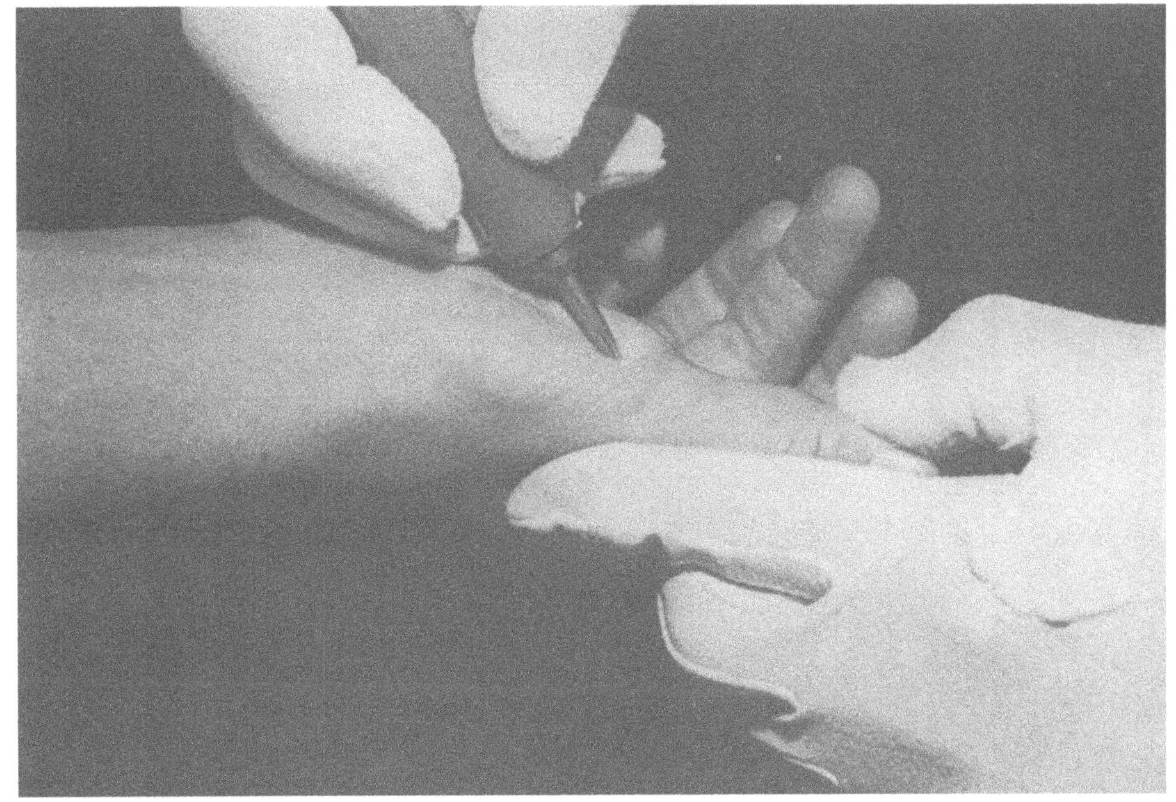

Lymph Drainage

6. MP-2a — Eye (eliminate toxins through organs first).

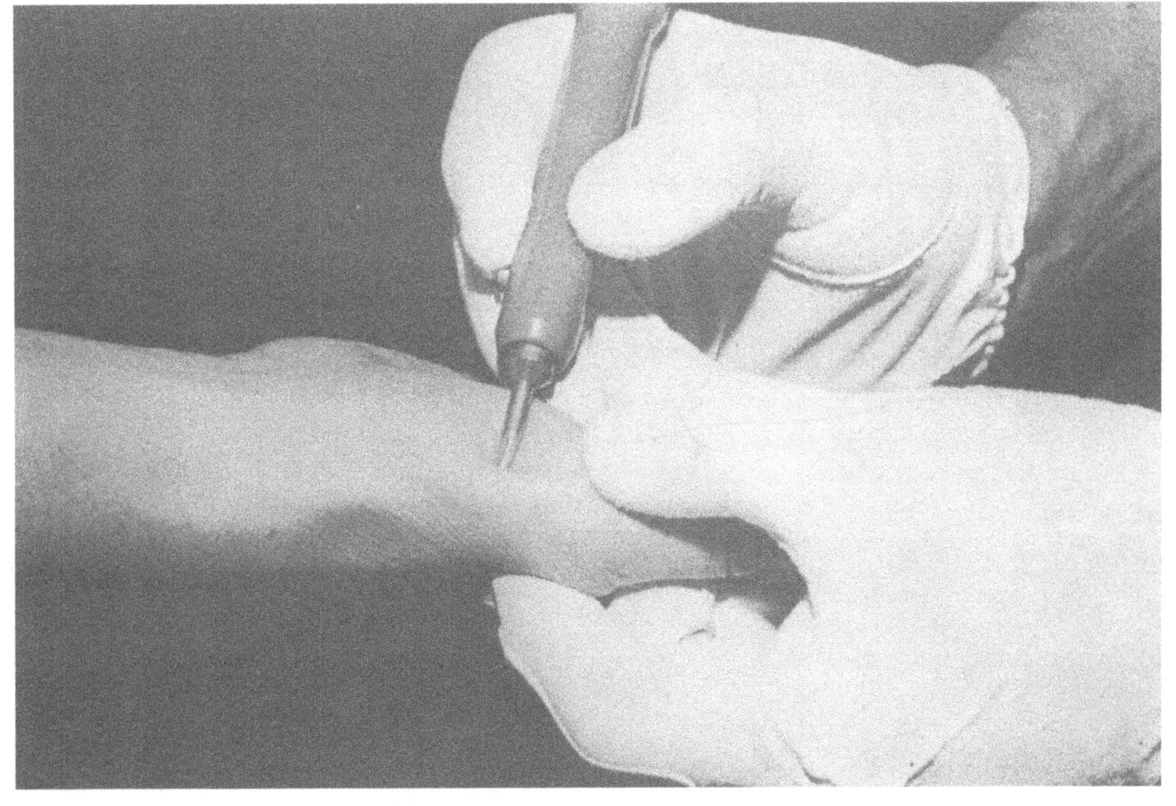

Lymph Drainage

7. MP-3 — Nose, paranasal sinus.

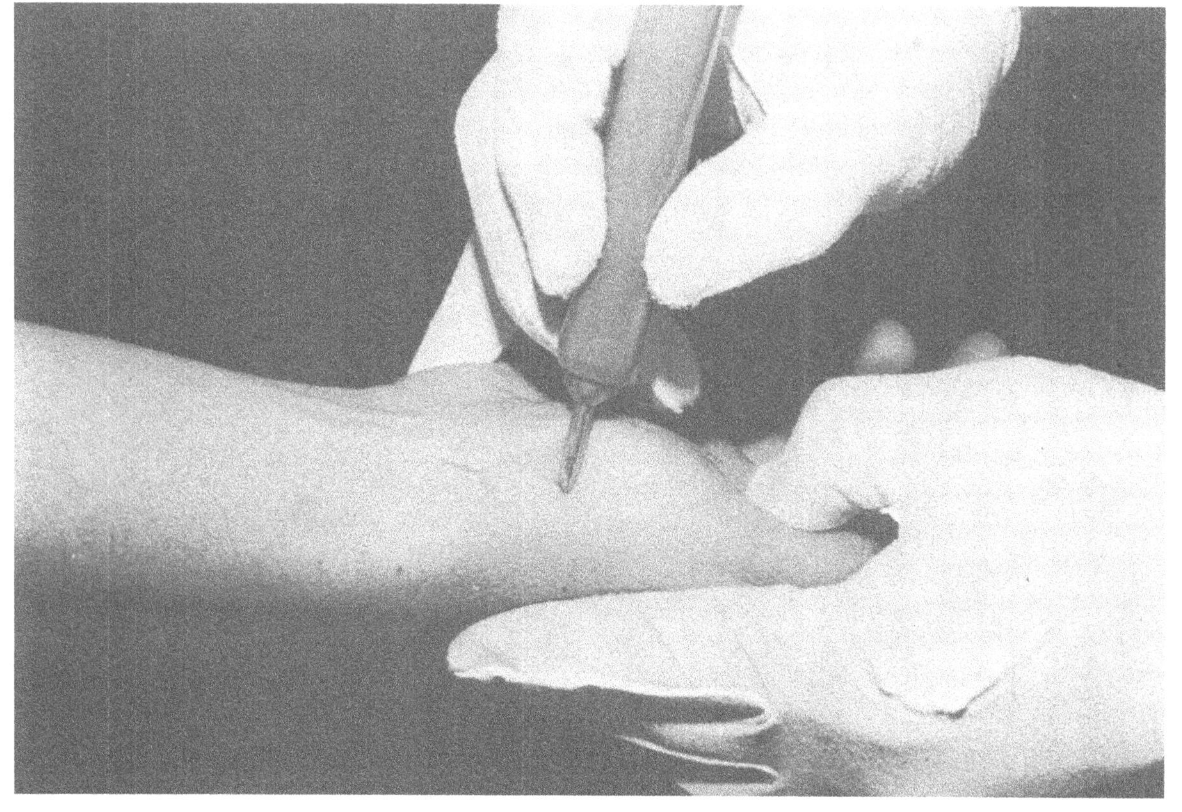

NOTES

Lung

Voll's *Illustrated Volume II,* fig. 17, p. 43.

1. MP-11—Alveoli of lung.
2. MP-10d — Mediastinal plexus (inhalants, hair dye, constant coughing, insecticides). (Right hand.)
3. CMP — Lower respiratory passage.
4. MP-10b — Bronchioli (emphysema, loss of elasticity of lung fibres).
5. MP-10a — Pleura (cancer, Hodgkin's Disease).
6. MP-10 — Bronchi (asthma).
7. MP-9a — Bronchial plexus.
8. MP-9 — Trachea.
9. MP-7 — Arteries of the upper extremities.
10. MP-8 — Veins of the upper extremities.
11. MP-8b — Larynx.
12. MP-8a — Hypopharynx.

NOTES

Lung

1. MP-11—Alveoli of lung.

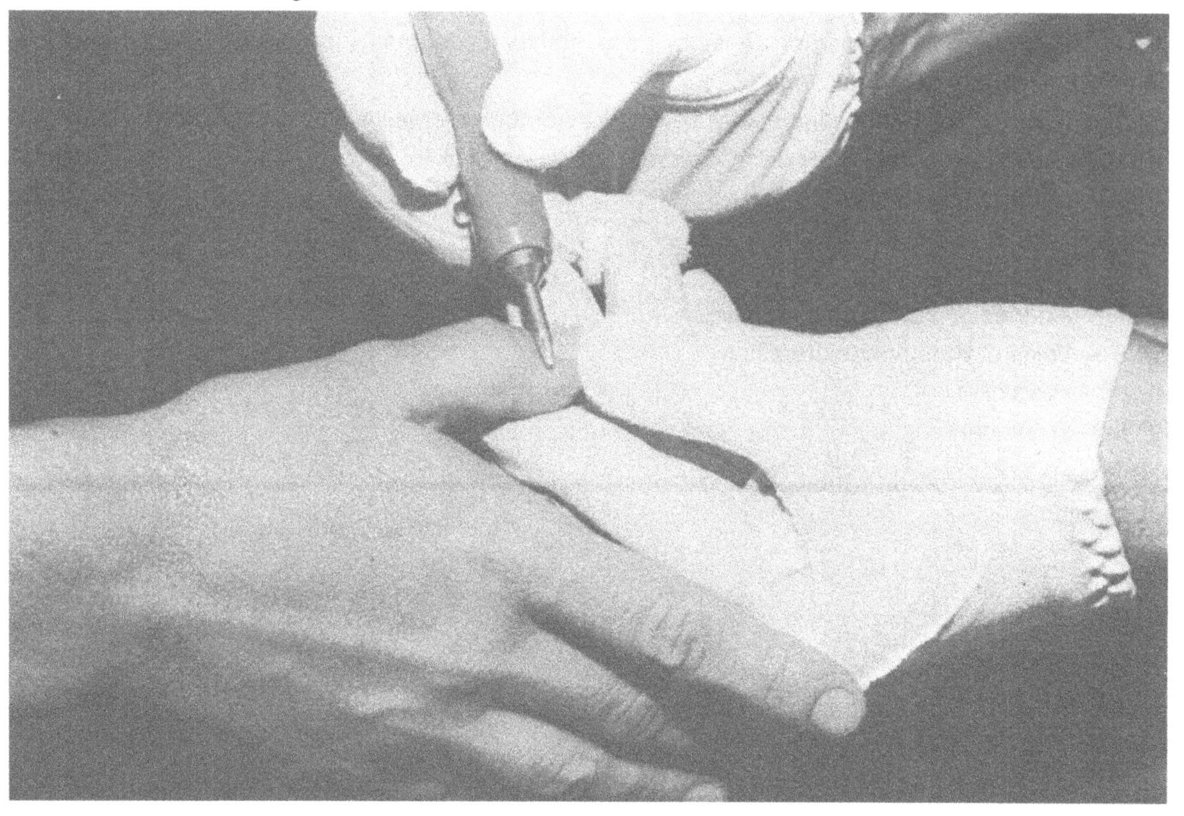

Lung

2. MP-10d — Mediastinal plexus (Right hand.)

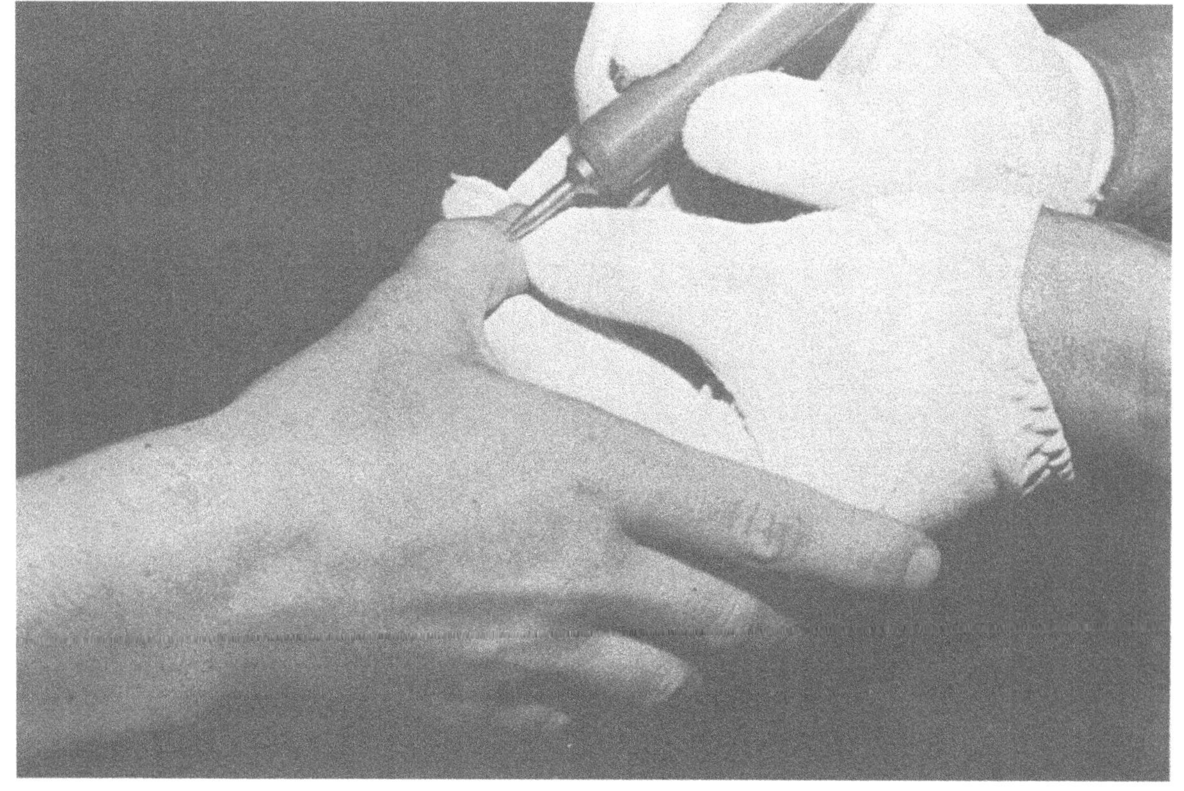

Lung
3. CMP — Lower respiratory passage.

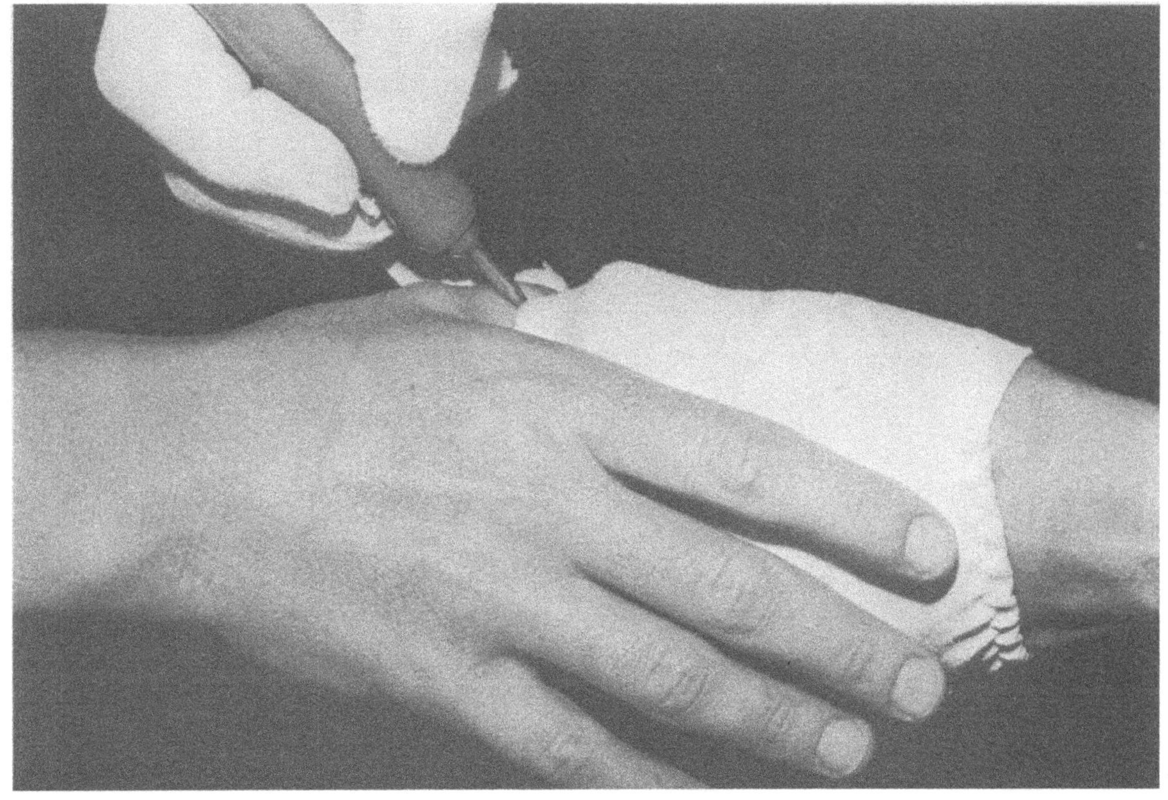

Lung
4. MP-10b — Bronchioli (emphysema, loss of elasticity of lung fibres).

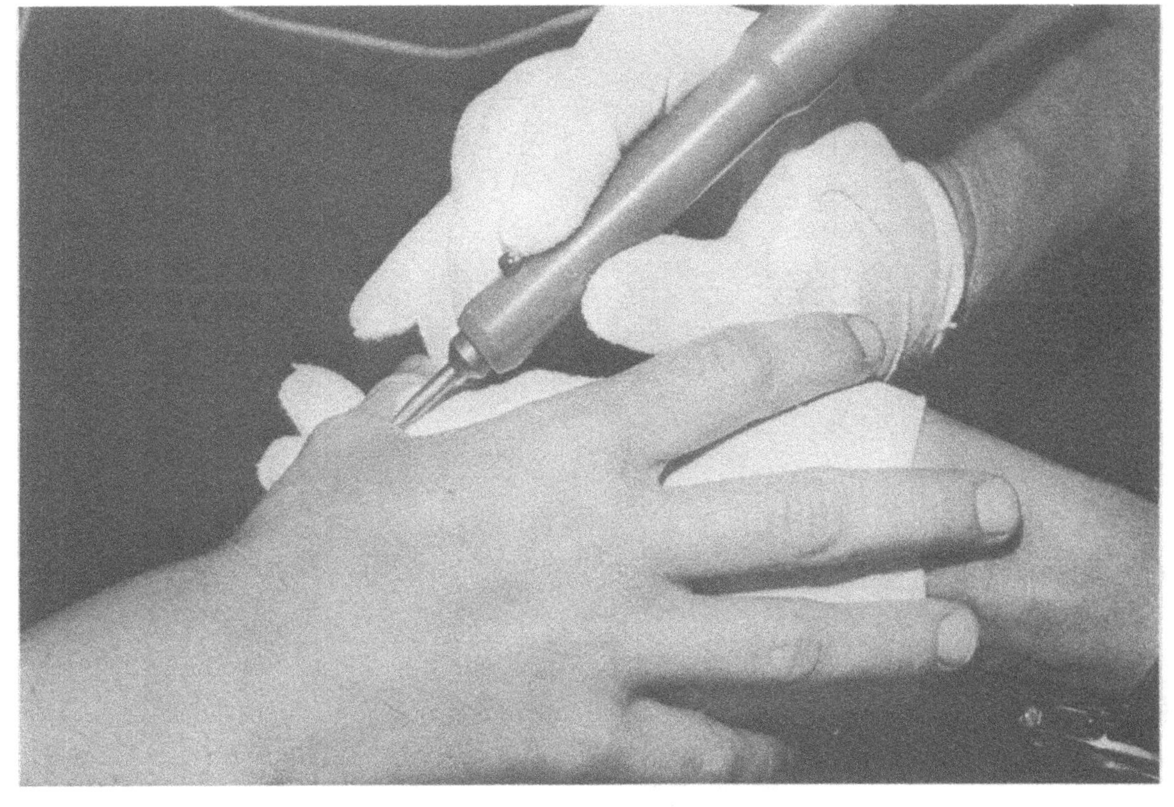

Lung

5. MP-10a — Pleura (cancer, Hodgkin's Disease).

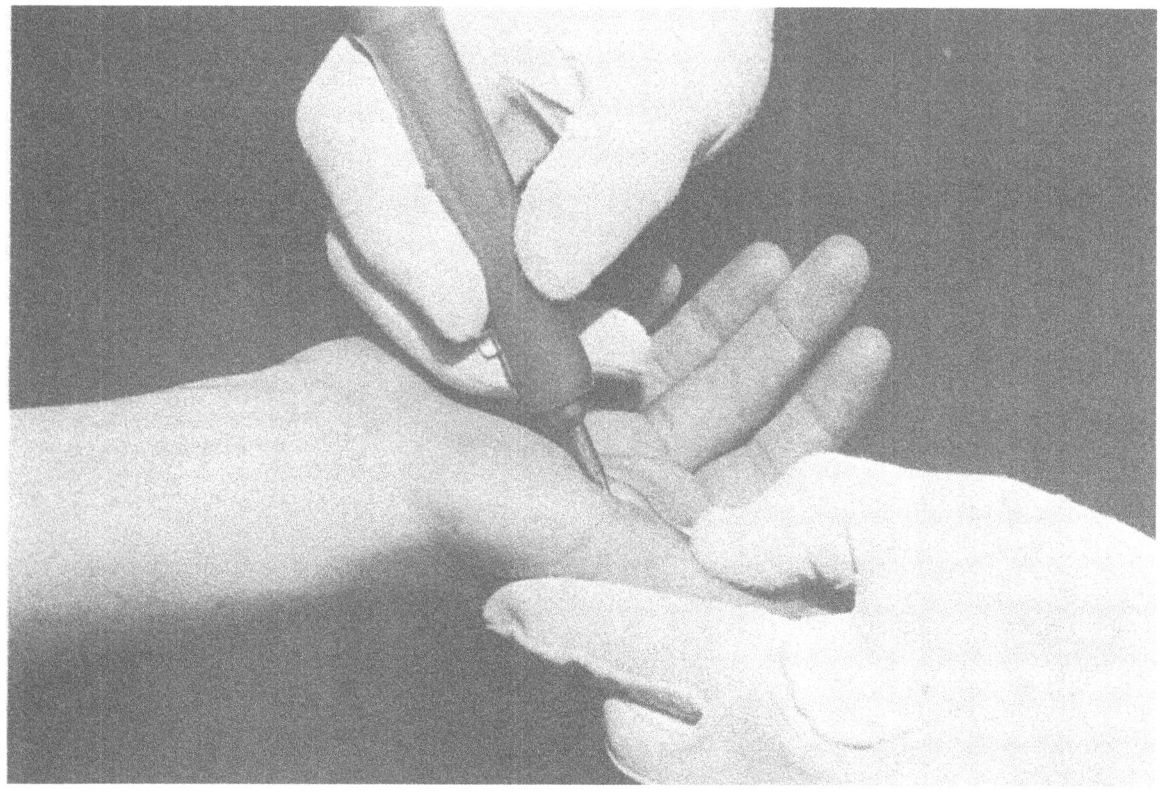

Lung

6. MP-10 — Bronchi (asthma).

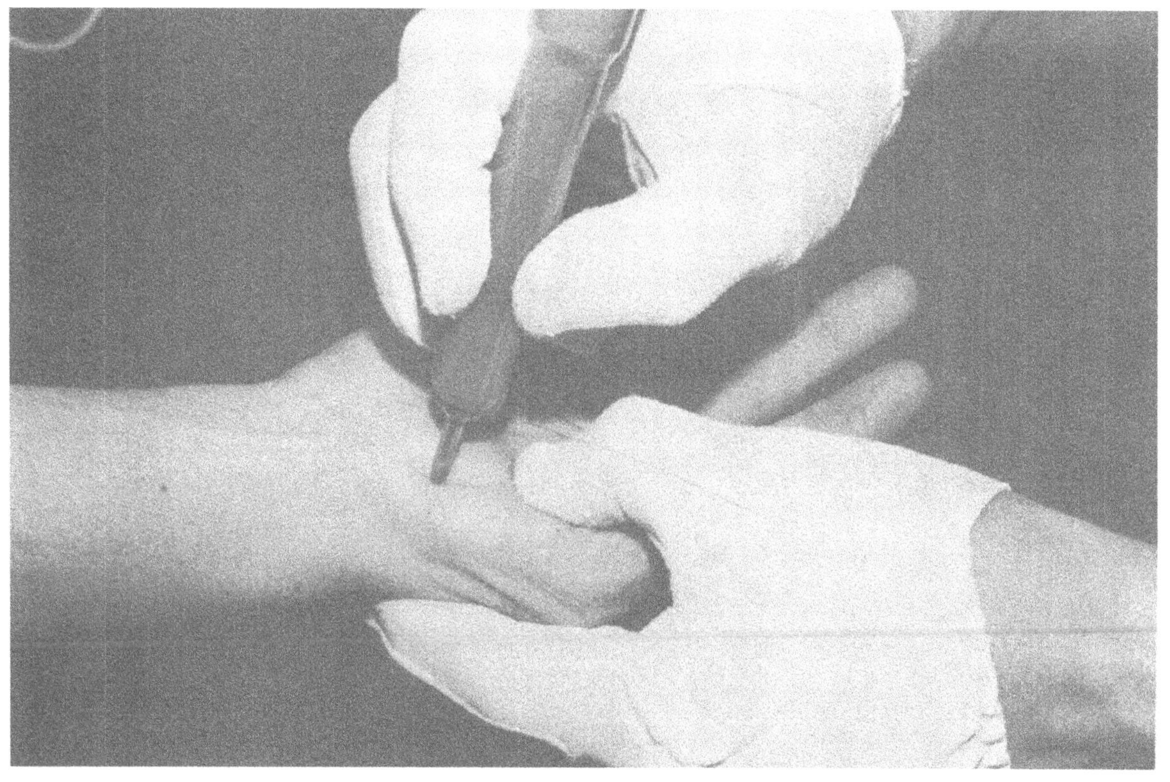

Lung Intestine

Voll's *Illustrated Volume II,* fig. 9, p. 27; fig. 10a, p. 28.
Intestinal auto-intoxication also affects heart.

RIGHT

1. MP-1 — Transverse colon, right.
2. MP-1a— Upper hypogastric plexus.
3. CMP.
4. MP —Peritoneum.
5. MP-2 — Hepatic flexure.
6. MP-3 — Ascending colon.
7. MP-4 — Coecum.
8. MP-4a— Appendix (chronic appendicitis — remote pain such as shoulder, thorax, coccyx disturbances, stomach malfunction and pain). Lymph nodes of ileo-cecal valve.
9. MP-19 —Nasal septum, lateral portion including conchae. (GV-23a — nasal cavity vault).
10. 10. MP-20 —Ethmoid cells.

LEFT

1. MP-1 — Sigmoid.

3. CMP.
4. MP — Peritoneum.
5. MP-2 — Descending colon.
6. MP-3 — Sigmoid flexure.
7. MP-4 — Transverse colon.
8. MP-4a — Mesentenal lymph nodes.

NOTES

Large Intestine

1. MP-1 —Transverse colon, right. 1. MP-1 —Sigmoid, left.

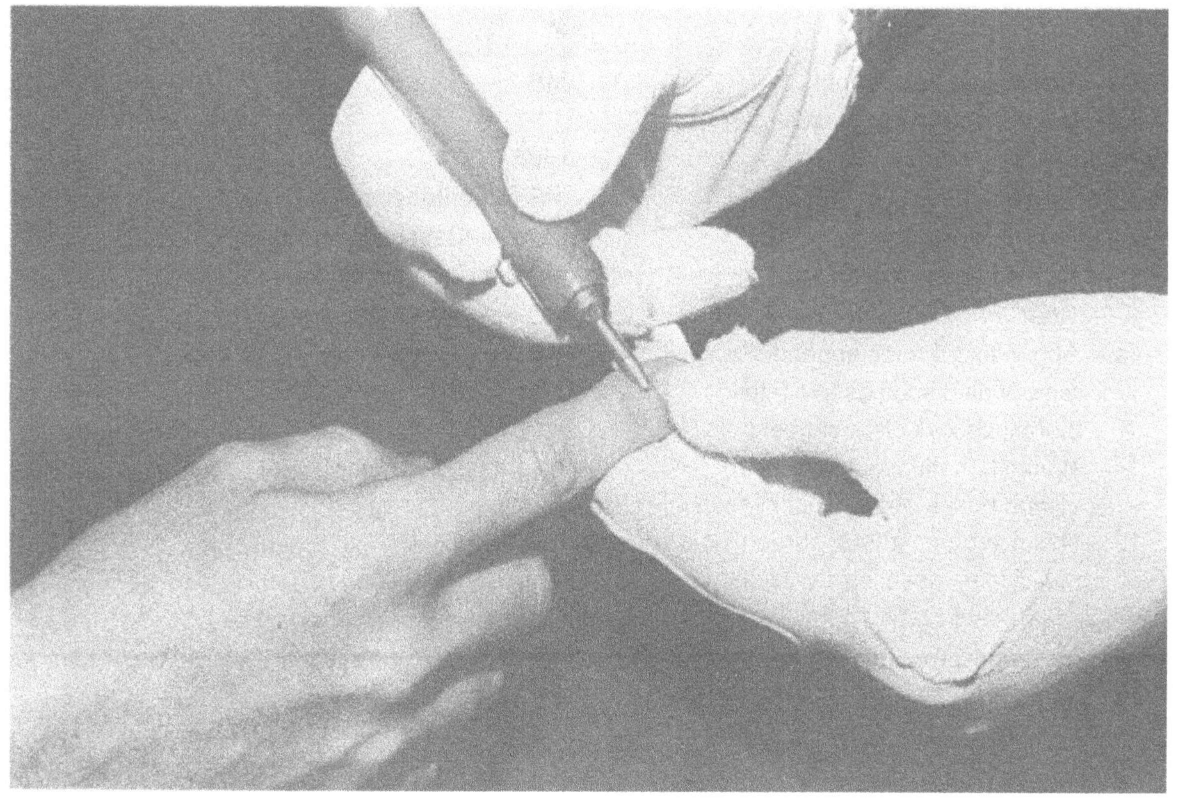

Large Intestine

3. CMP. 3. CMP.

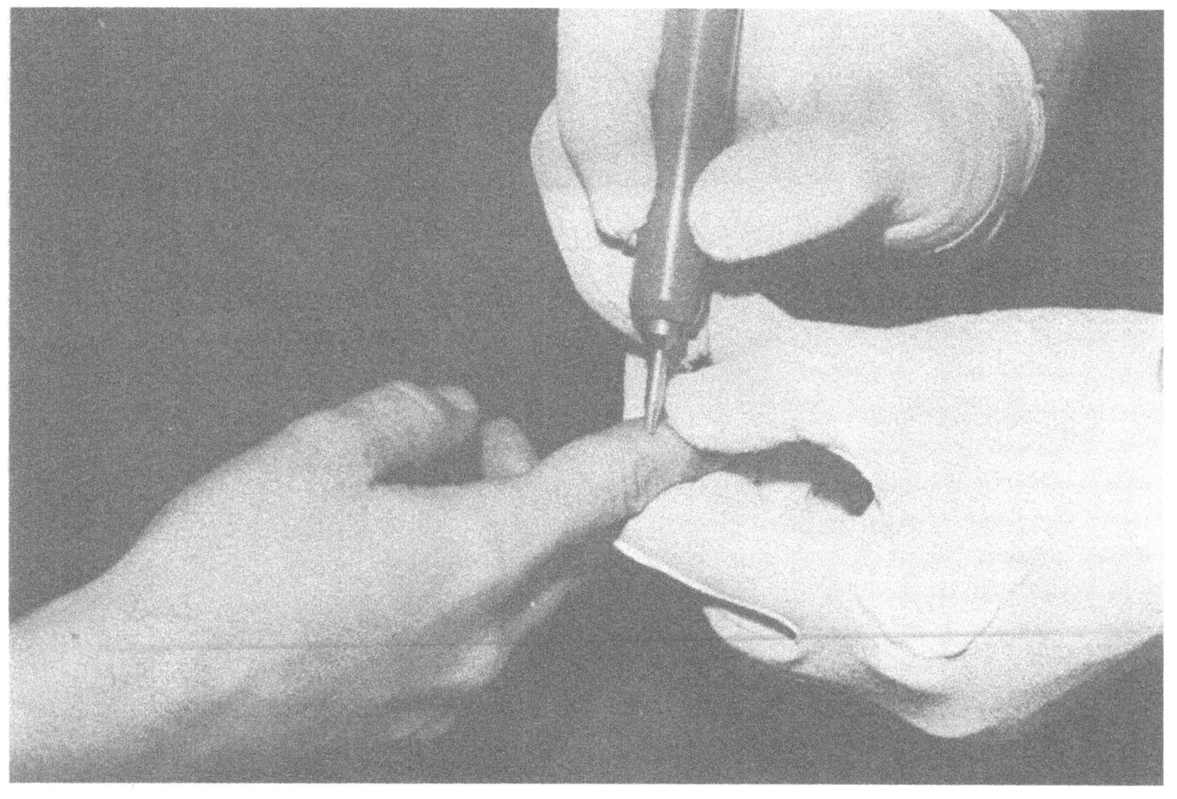

Large Intestine

4. MP — Peritoneum, right. 4. MP — Peritoneum, left.

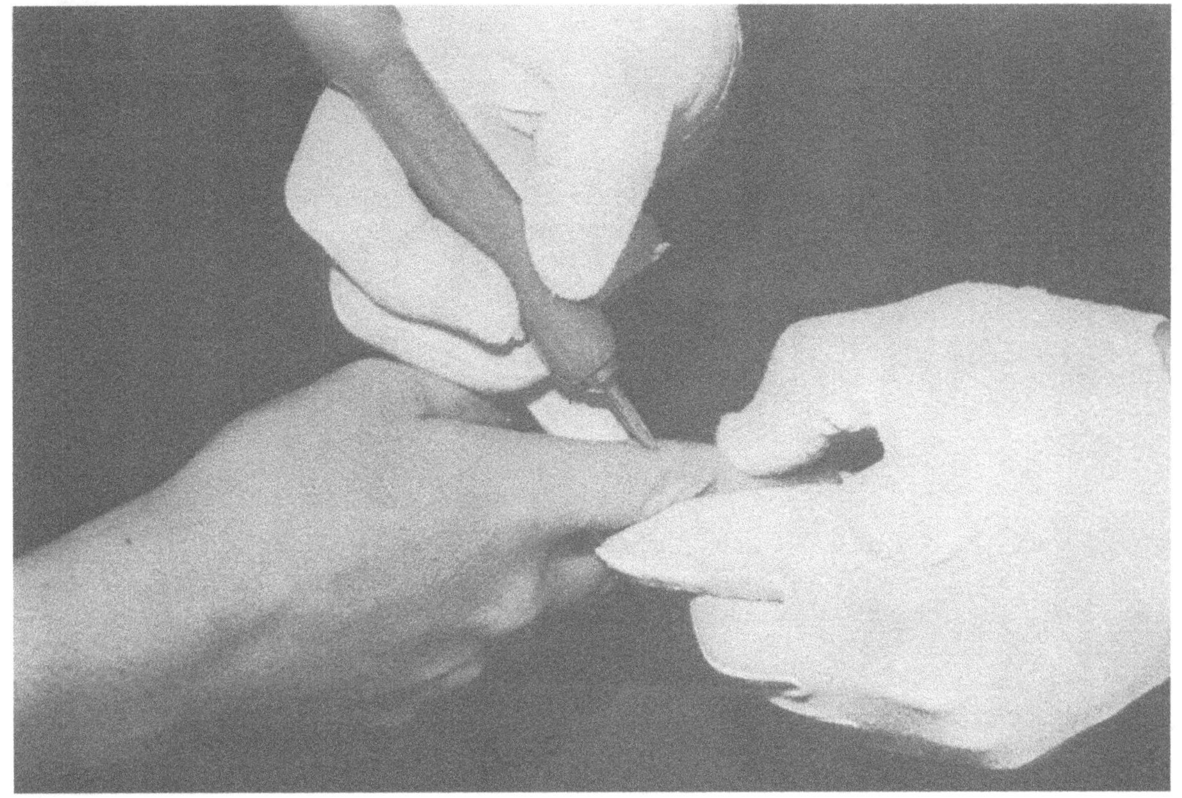

Large Intestine

5. MP-2 — Hepatic flexure, right. 5. MP-2 Descending colon, left.

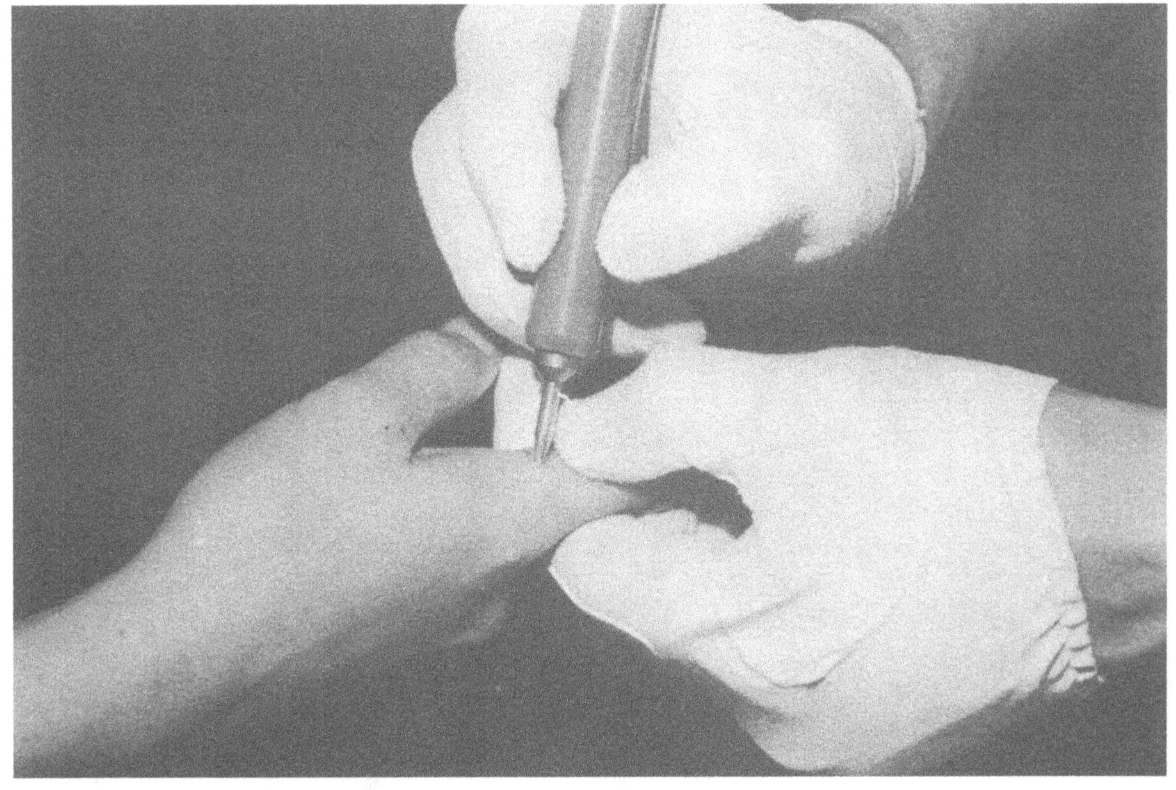

Large Intestine

6. MP-3 — Ascending colon, right. 6. MP-3 — Sigmoid flexure, left.

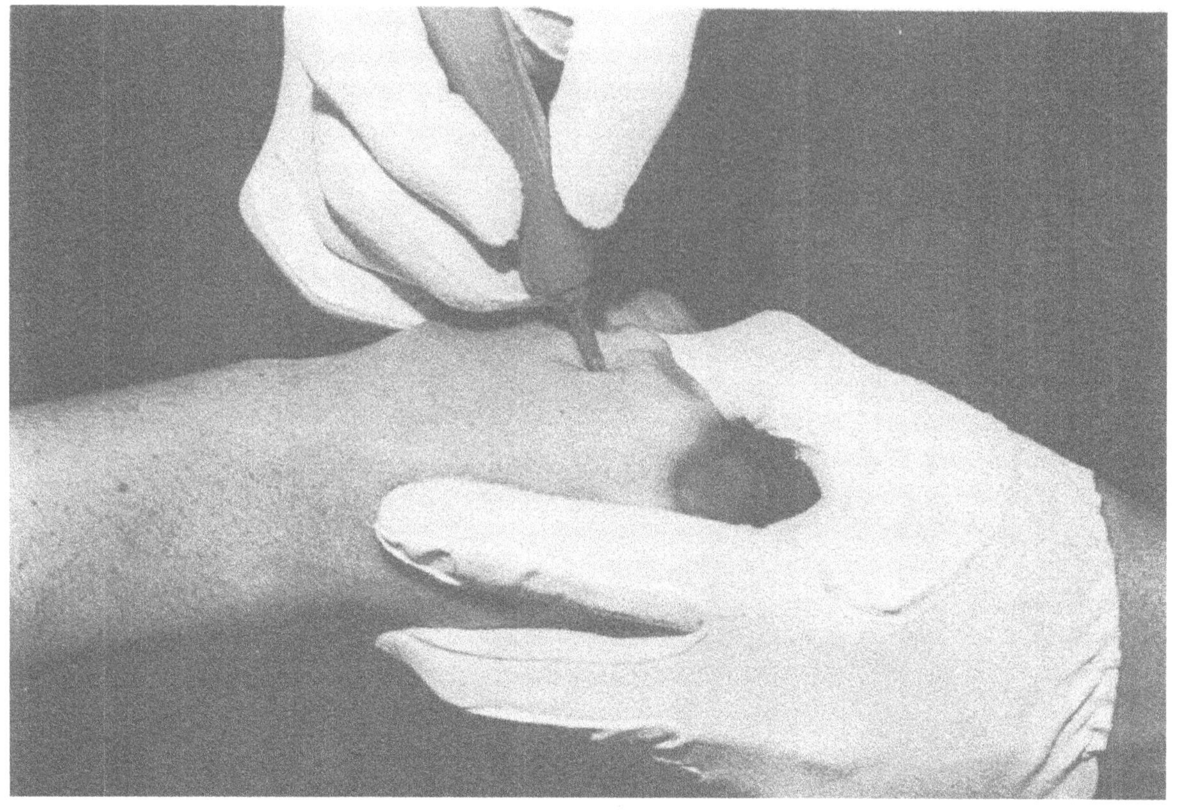

Large Intestine

7. MP-4 —Coecum, right. 7. MP-4 — Transverse colon, left.

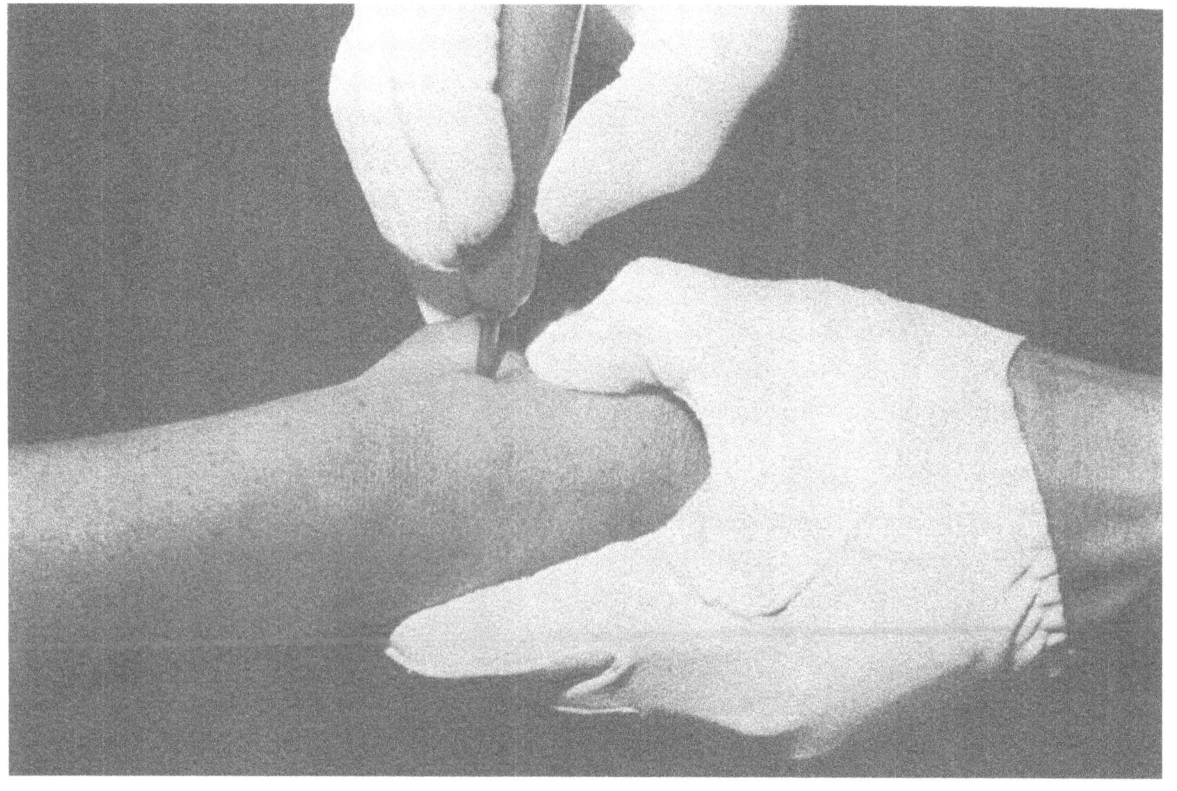

Large Intestine

8. MP-4a— Appendix (chronic appendicitis, right. 8. MP-4a—Mesentenal lymph nodes, left.

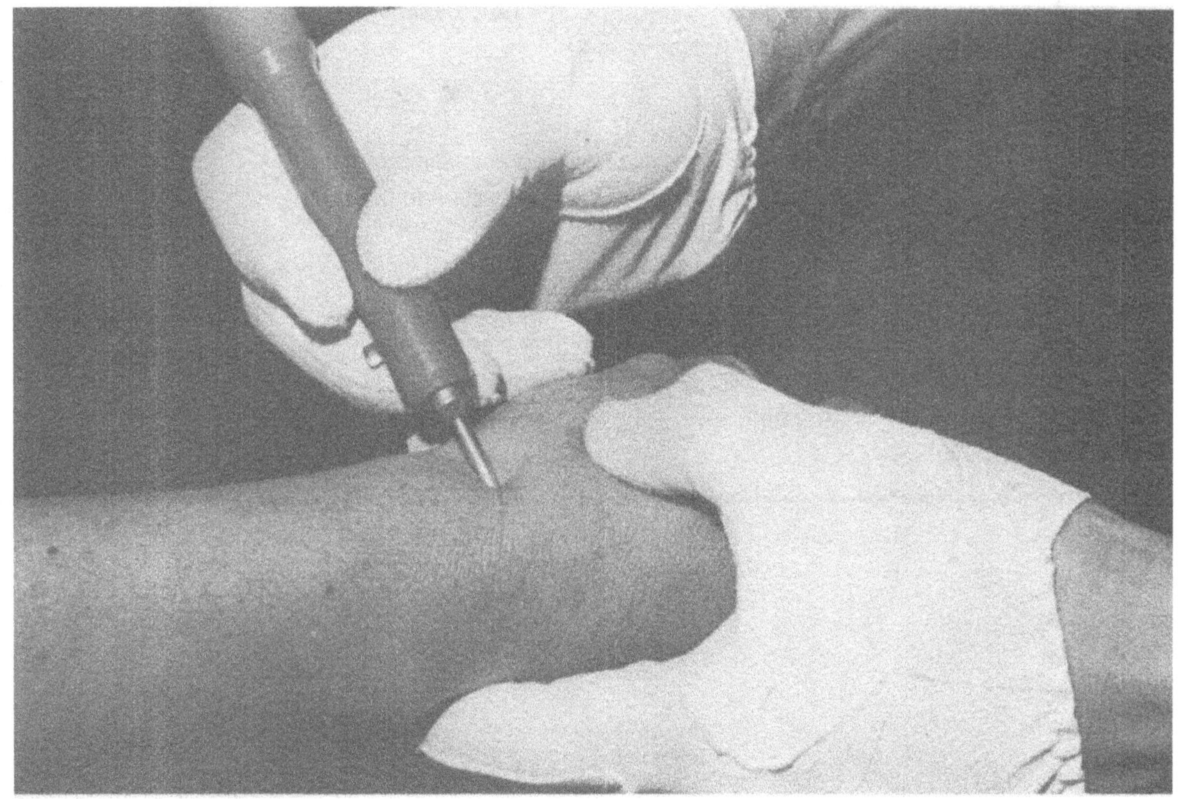

NOTES

Nerve Degeneration (Tri-part div.)

Voll's *Illustrated Volume II,* fig. 33, p. 75.

1. MP-1 — Lumbar and sacral marrow, lower part of body, lumbarsacral plexus.
2. MP-1a — Autonomic nervous system including vagus.
3. CMP.
4. MP-1 -2 — Meninges and spinal marrow.
5. MP-2 — Cervical and thoracic plexuses, cervical and thoracic spine marrow.
6. MP-3 — Brain stem and cerebrum (stroke, marrow degeneration in the brain).
7. MP-3a — Parasympathetic cranial ganglia.
    a. GBL-MP-1a — Ciliary ganglion (eye problem).
    b. Secondary vessel point — MP-pterygopalatine ganglion (whole vegetative steering of the mouth vault, parts of the jaw, sensations in the mouth).
    c. SI-MP-18a —Otic ganglion.
    d. St-MP-8-3 — Submandibular ganglion (excess saliva).
8. MP-4 — Cranial nerves.

NOTES

Nerve Degeneration

1. MP-1 — Lumbar and sacral marrow, lower part of body, lumbarsacral plexus.

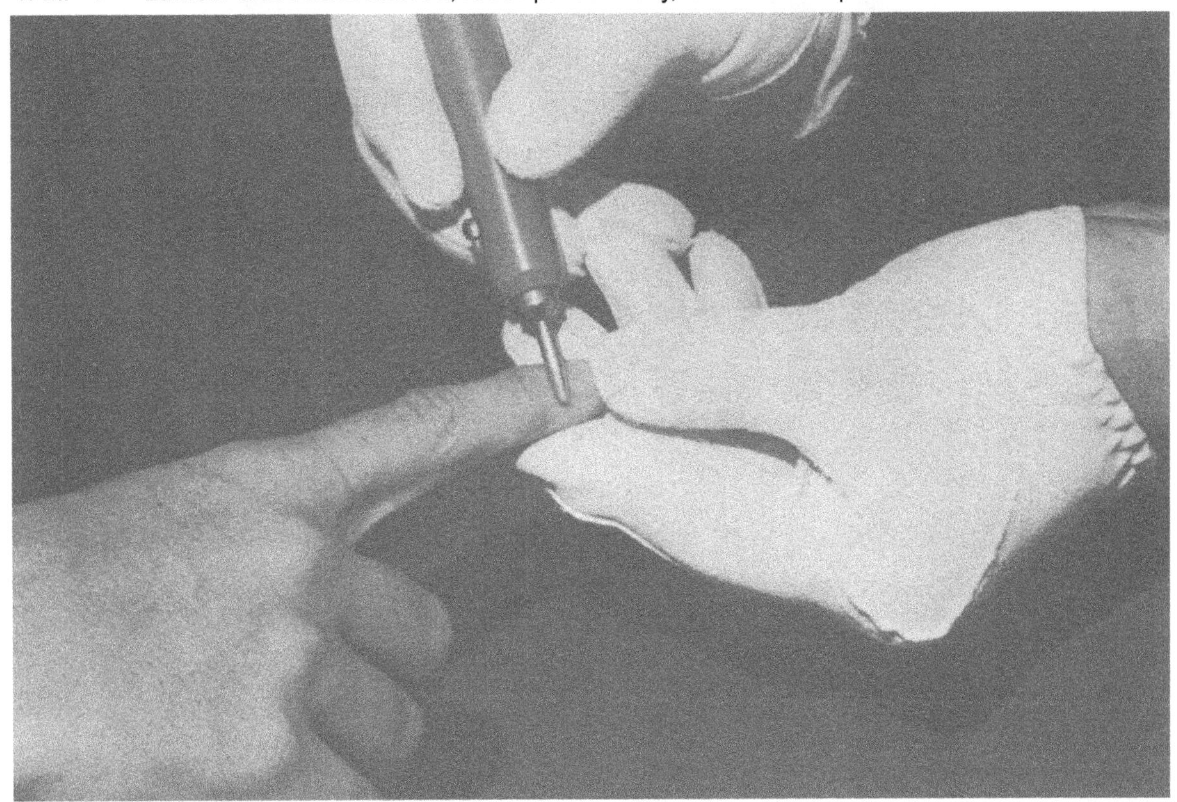

Nerve Degeneration

2. MP-1a — Autonomic nervous system including vagus.

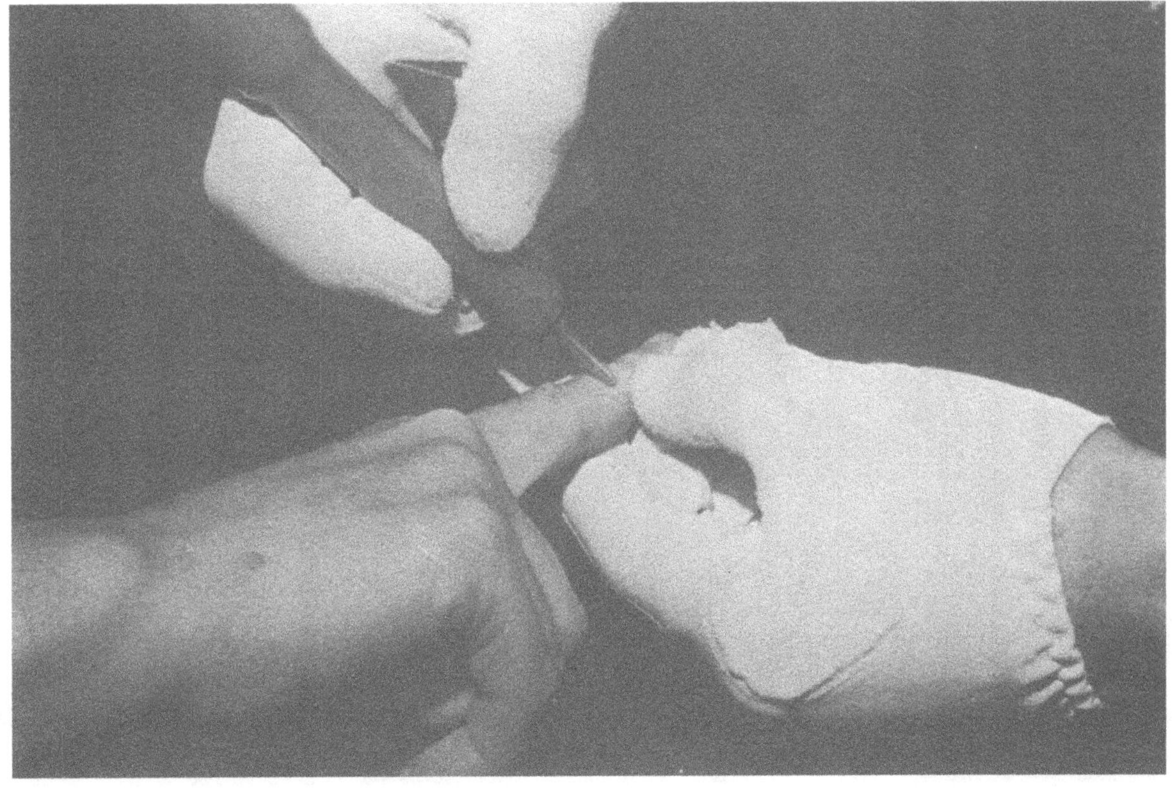

Nerve Degeneration
3. CMP.

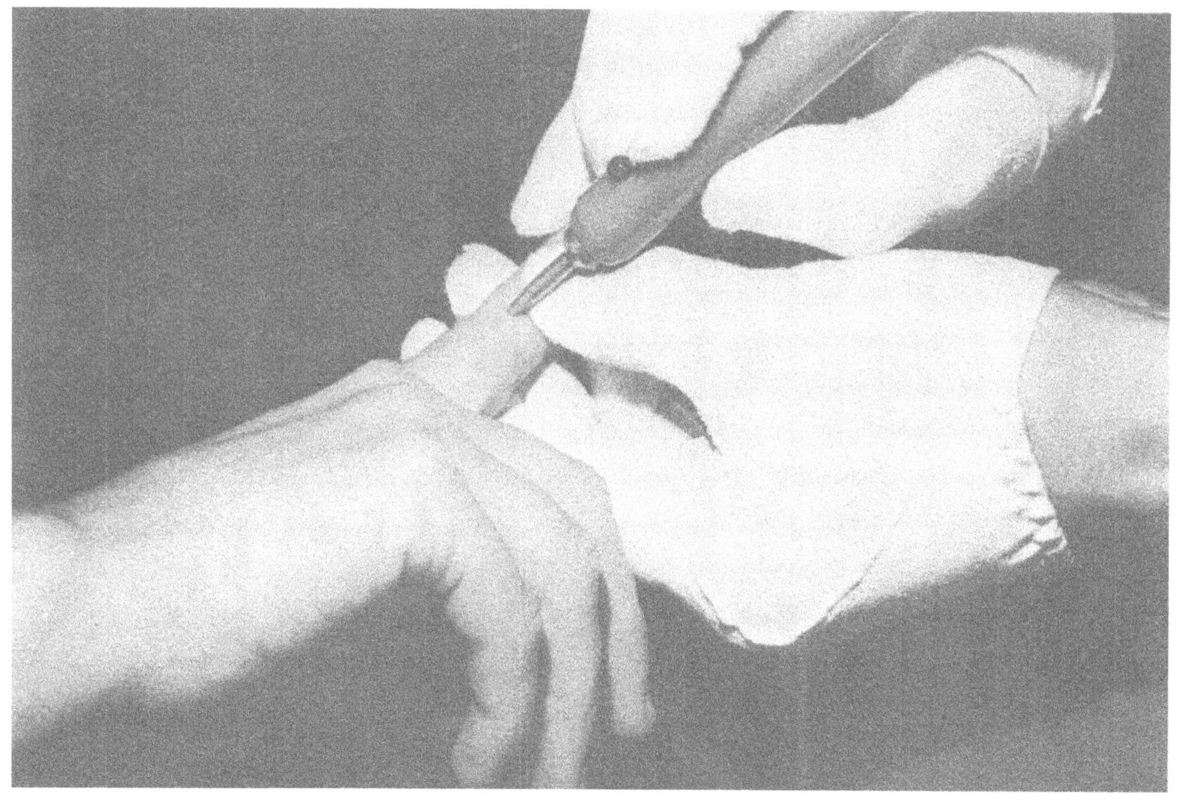

Nerve Degeneration
4. MP-1-2 — Meninges and spinal marrow

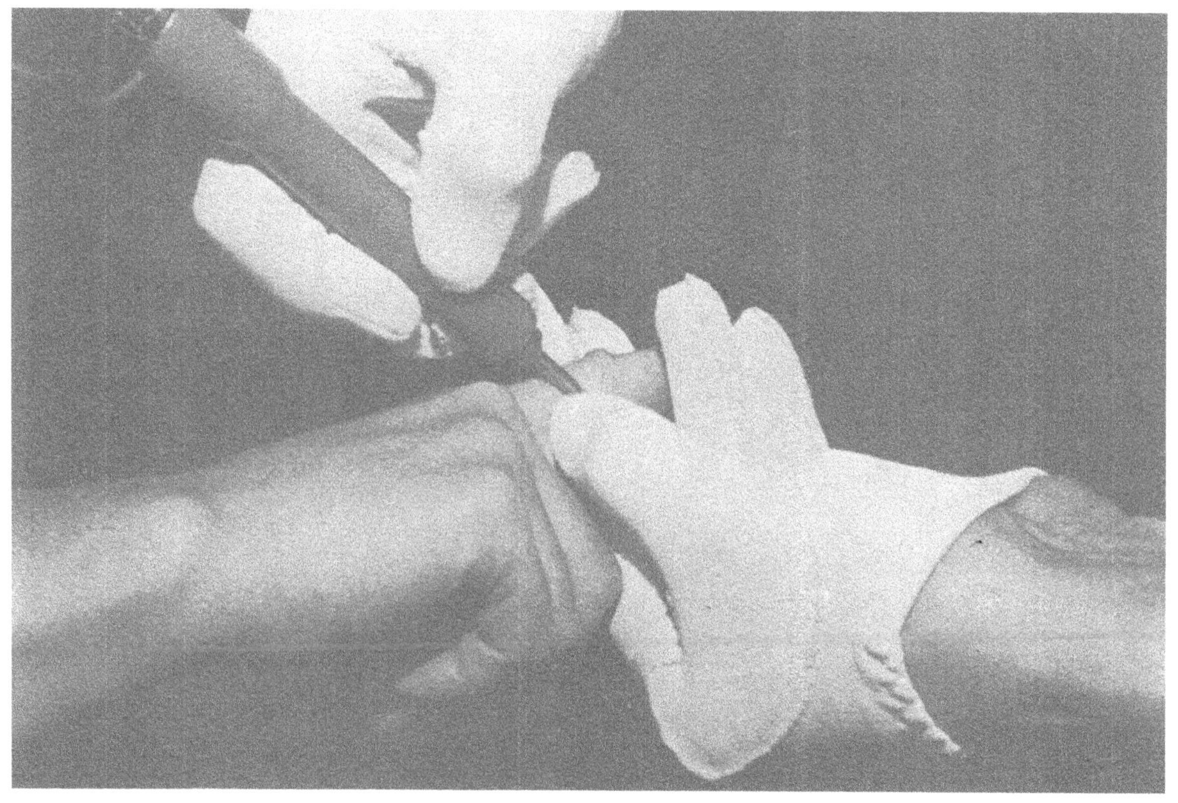

Nerve Degeneration

5. MP-2 — Cervical and thoracic plexuses, cervical and thoracic spine marrow..

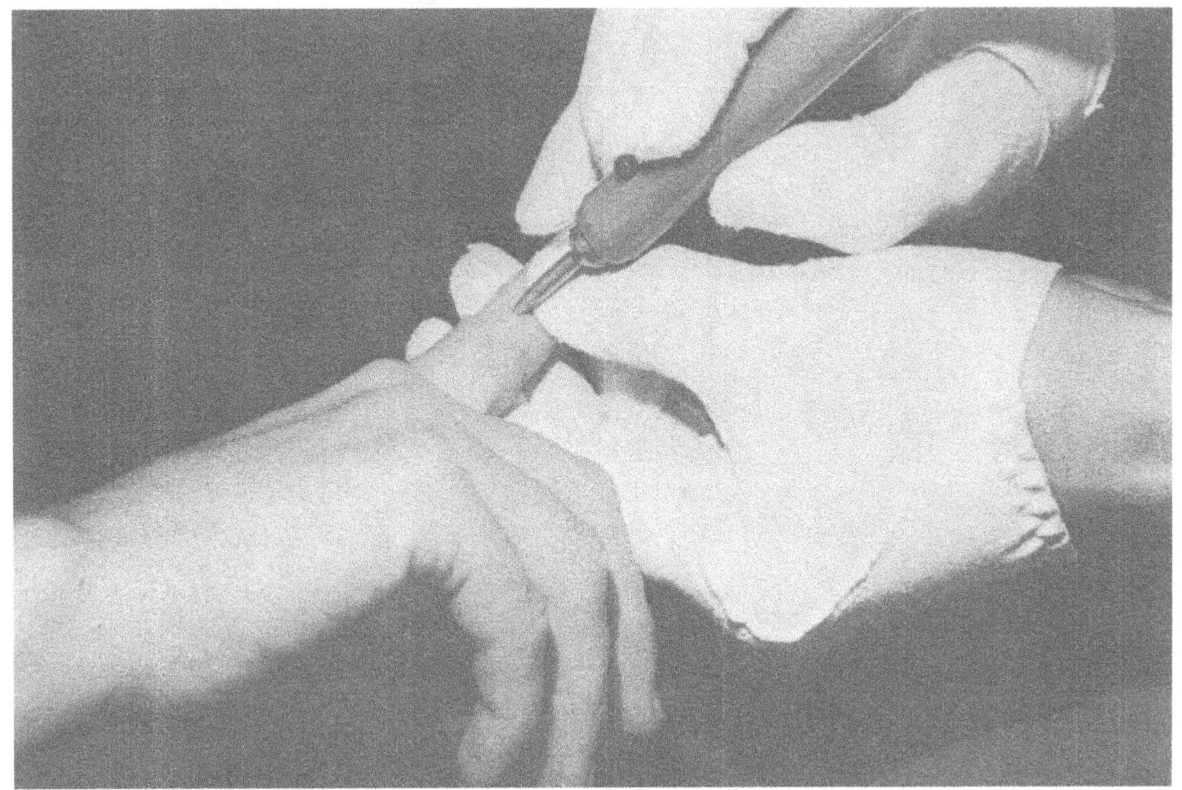

Nerve Degeneration

6. MP-3 — Brain stem and cerebrum (stroke, marrow degeneration in the brain).

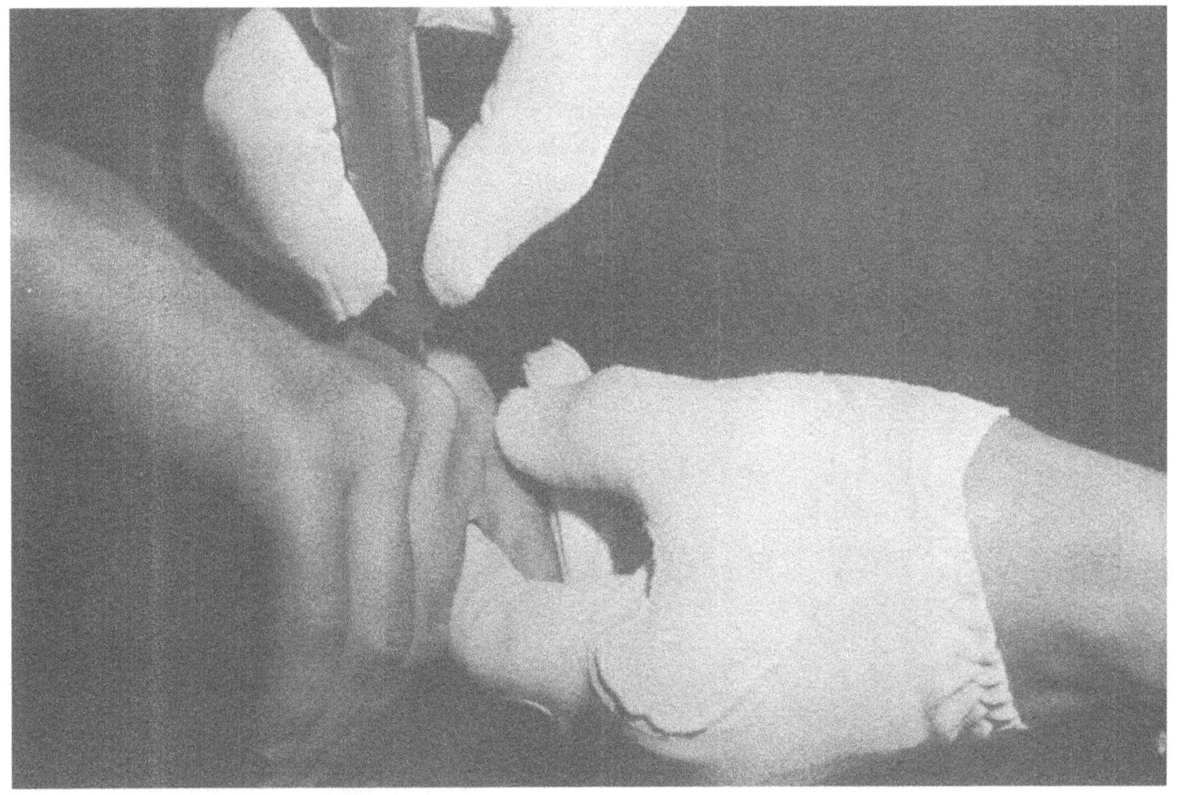

Nerve Degeneration

7. MP-3a — Parasympathetic cranial ganglia.

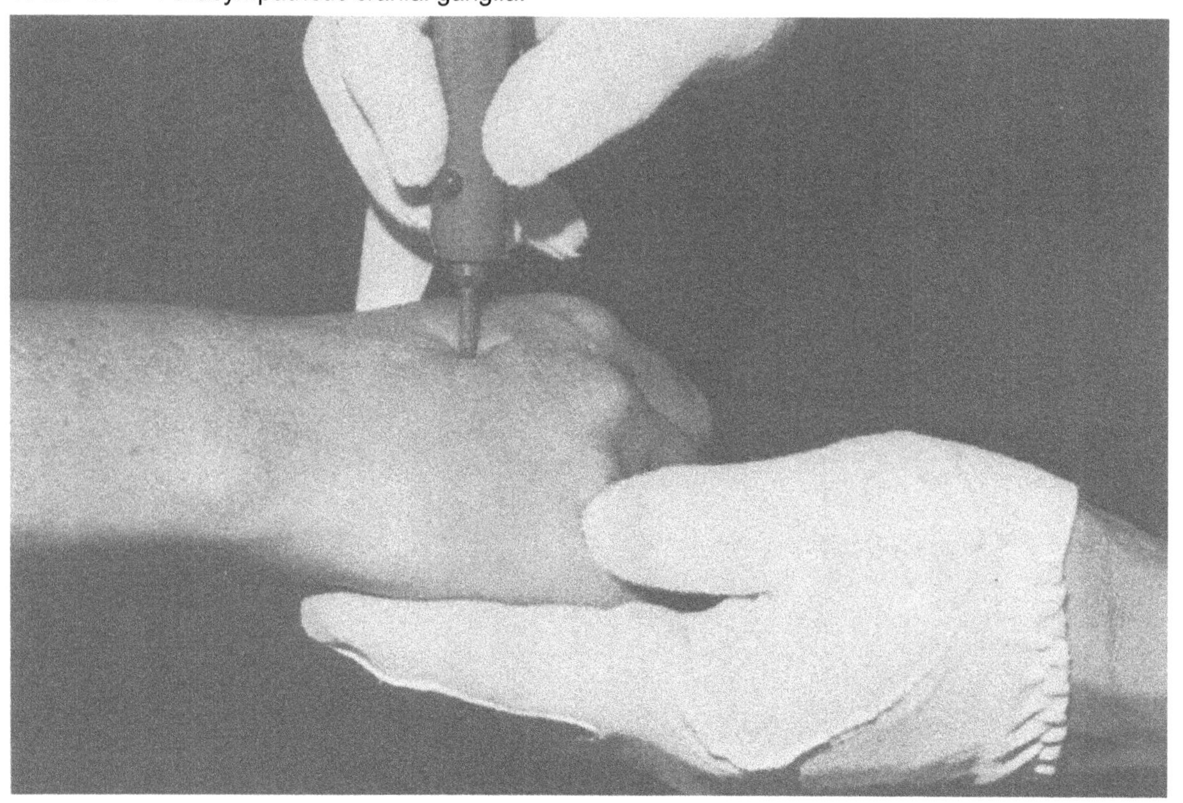

Nerve Degeneration

8. MP-4 — Cranial nerves.

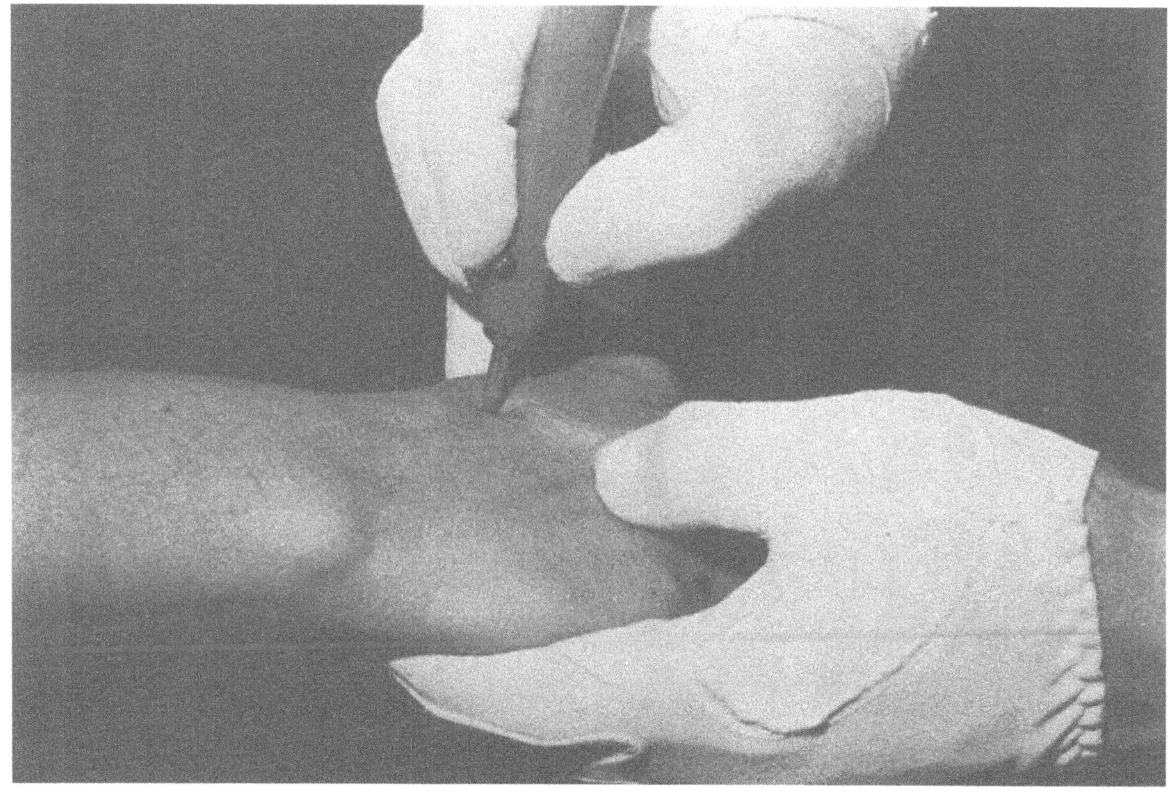

Circulation

Voll's *Illustrated Volume II,* fig. 2, p. 13.

1. MP-9 — Arteries on same side upper and lower, Lu-7 arteries of upper extremities, St-32 arteries of leg.
2. MP-8e— Cardiac ganglia (right hand), thoracic aortic plexus (left hand).
3. CMP—Dorsal side.
4. MP-8c — Abdominal aortic plexus (right hand), abdominal aorta (left hand). Palm side.
5. MP-8b — Cisterna chyli, in case of ID on CMP peritoneum LI, peritoneum ileum and duodenum — hand; fibroid degeneration peritoneum — peritoneum Pa, peritoneum Li, peritoneum St, peritoneum GBL, peritoneum Ki, peritoneum UBL, genito-urinary organs — foot. Cisterna chyli covers all lymphatics. Dorsal side.
6. MP-8a — Thoracic duct (lower part of the lymph) (right hand). Blockage in thoracic duct has pain and tenderness in Ki-27, St-43. Left hand — accessory thoracic duct. Palm side.
7. MP-8 — Veins on same side (palm side MP) (varicose veins, Lu-8 veins of the upper extremity, Pa-Sp-10 pelvic veins, St-33 abdominal veins, Li-7 — veins of lower extremities). Palm side.
8. MP-8d — Aortic arch (right hand), thoracic aorta (left hand). Dorsal side.
9. MP-Lymph — System ID from 90 to 70 may be a degenerative illness of the lymph system, like leukemia.
10. MP-7 — Coronary vessels (palm side MP) at wrist.
11. MP-7a — Coronary plexus of heart.
12. MP-Heart MP-6 — Heart muscle, at wrist.
13. MP-3 —Elbow joint 2nd MP.
14. MP-2 —Shoulder —arm joint 2nd MP.

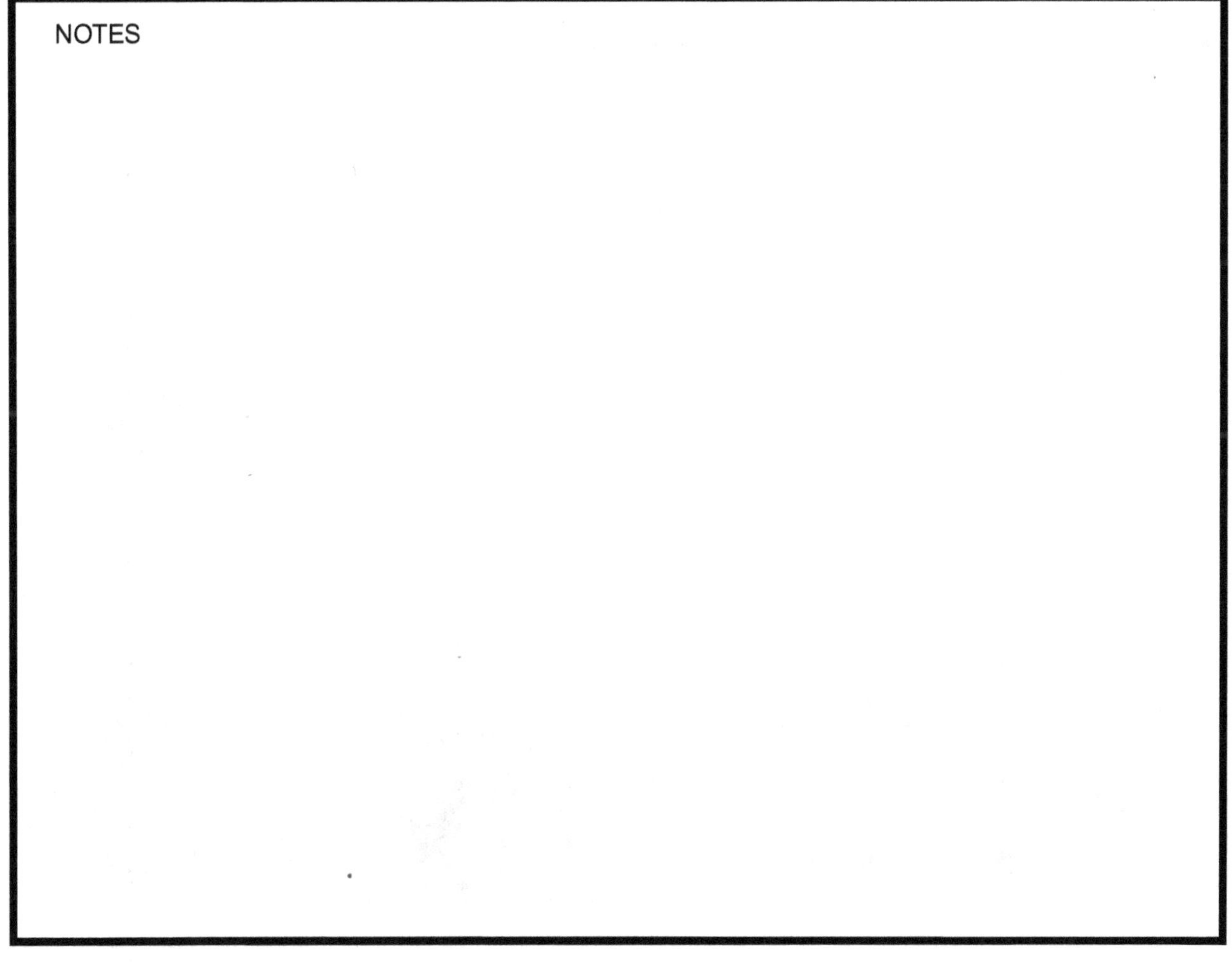

Circulation

1. MP-9 —Arteries.

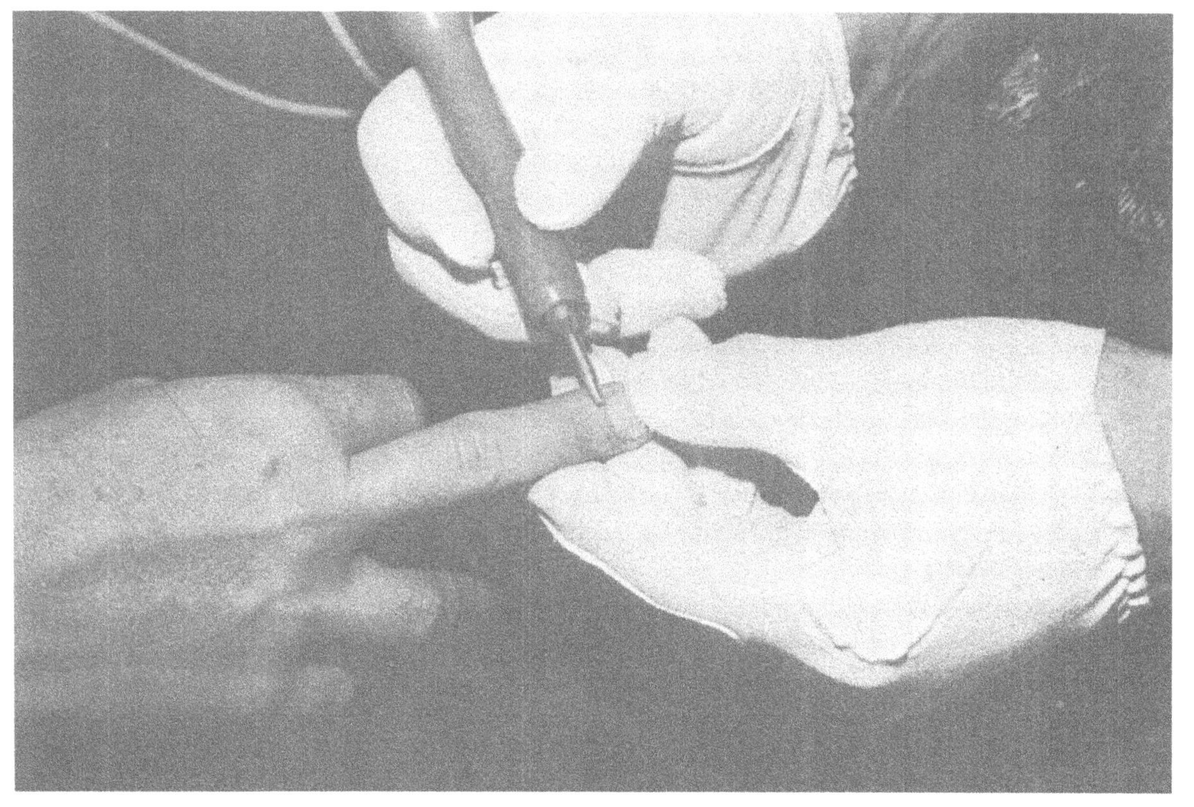

Circulation

3. CMP —Dorsal side.

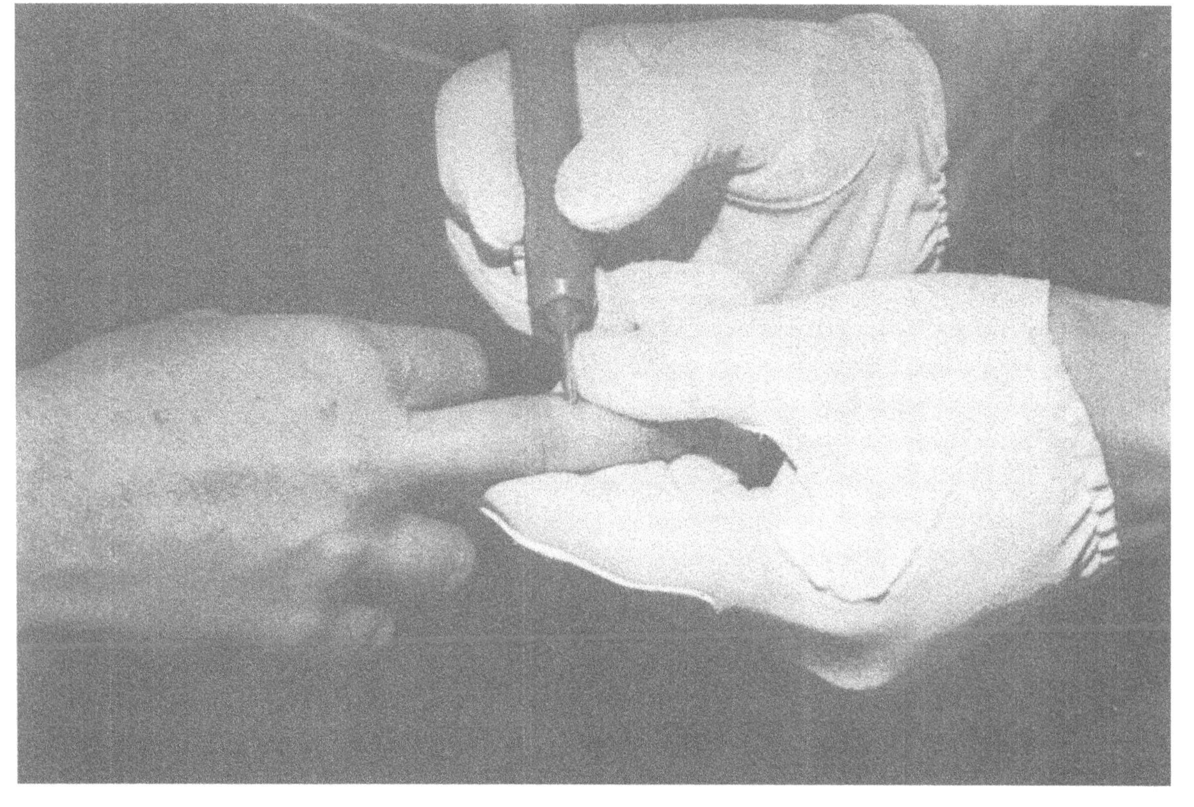

Circulation

7. MP-8 — Veins on same side (palm side MP) (varicose veins).

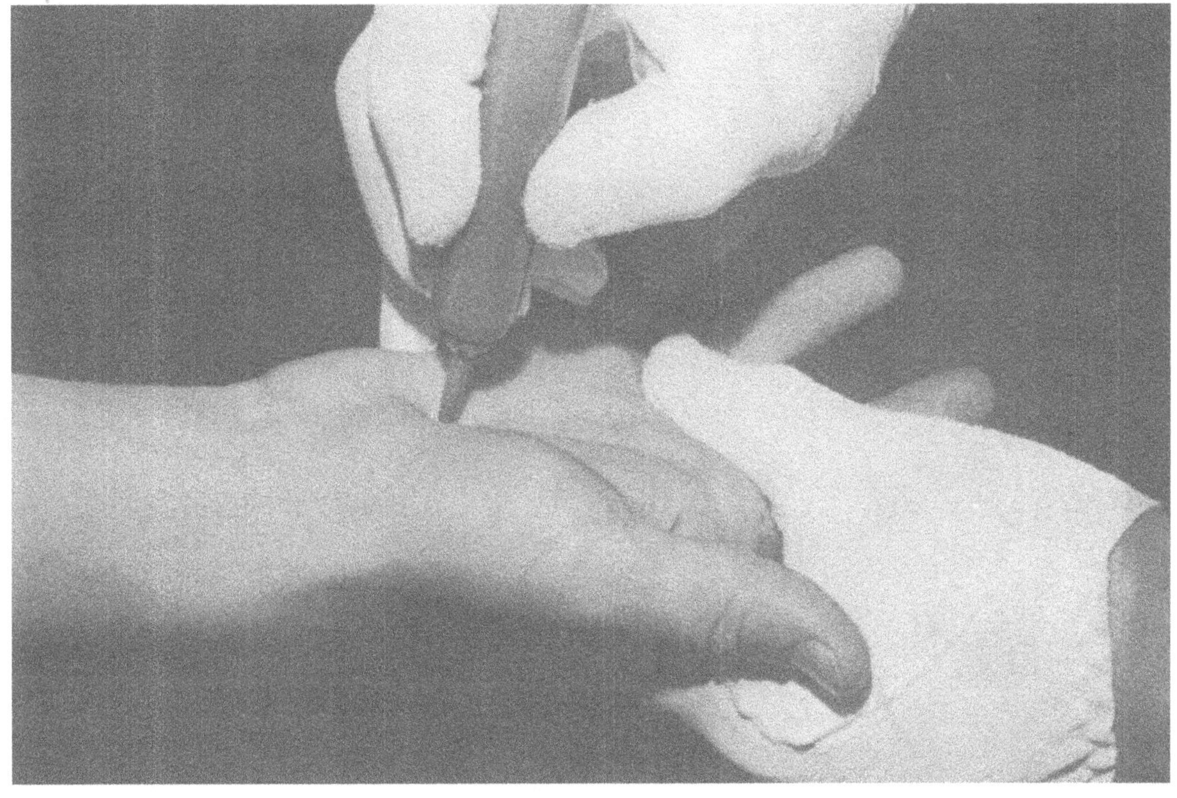

Circulation

9. MP-Lymph.

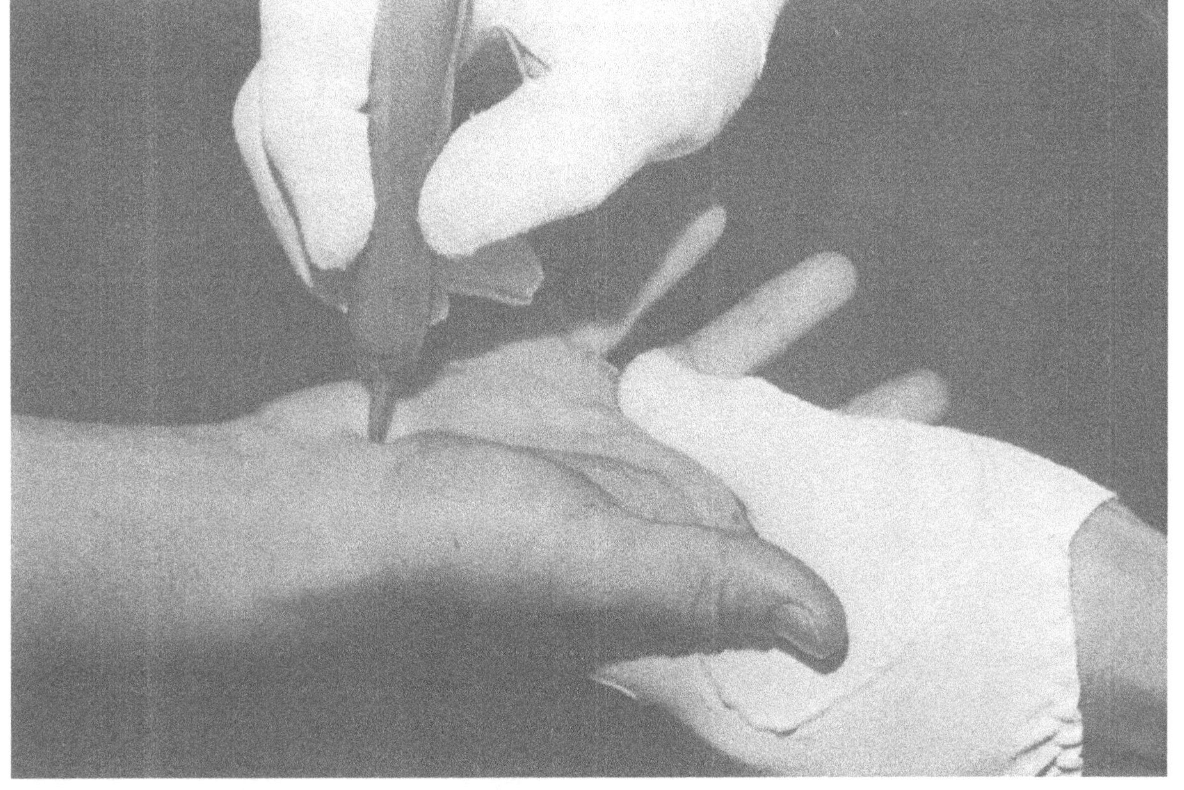

Circulation

10. MP-7 — Coronary vessels (palm side MP) at wrist.

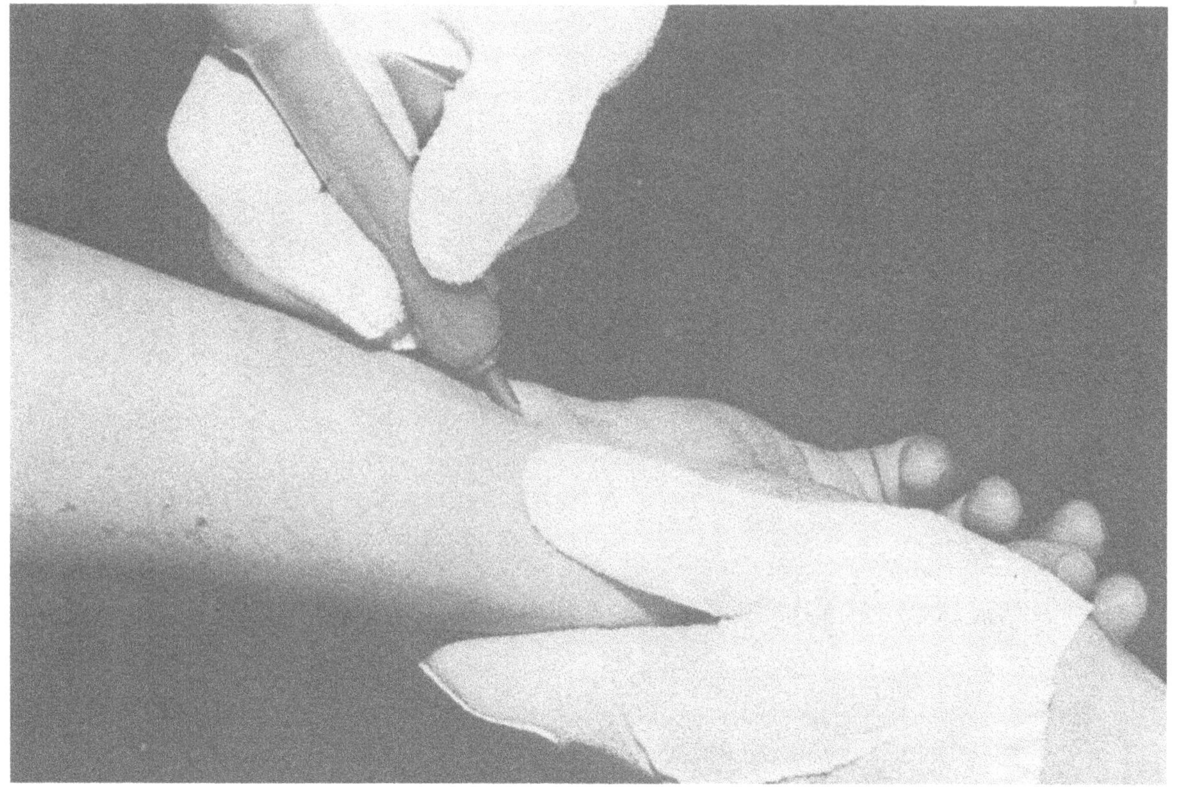

NOTES

Allergy

Voll's *Illustrated Volume II,*fig. 21, p. 51.

Check spleen, damaged liver.

1. MP-1 — Skin of lower portion, lower extremities, abdominals and minor pelvis (allergy caused by insecticides, intestinal, food, food coloring).
2. CMP —Allergy.
3. Vascular sclerosis — Arteriosclerosis (check coronary vessel MP-7; brain-nerve degeneration MP-3; Ki-3 arterial and arteriolar sclerotic changes in kidney and glomerulo-sclerosis). Sedate vascular sclerosis to 50, if others above are affected at least 10 points, use iodine type of medicine.
4. MP-2 — Skin of upper portion of the body — thoracic, neck, nape, upper extremities, allergy of organs in the chest (inhalant, respiration problems).
5. MP-3 — Skin of the head, allergies of organs of the head, oral cavity, nasal and paranasal sinus (trigeminal neuralgia, dental materials 90, 92, drippy nose, toothache point).

NOTES

Allergy

1. MP-1—Skin of lower portion.

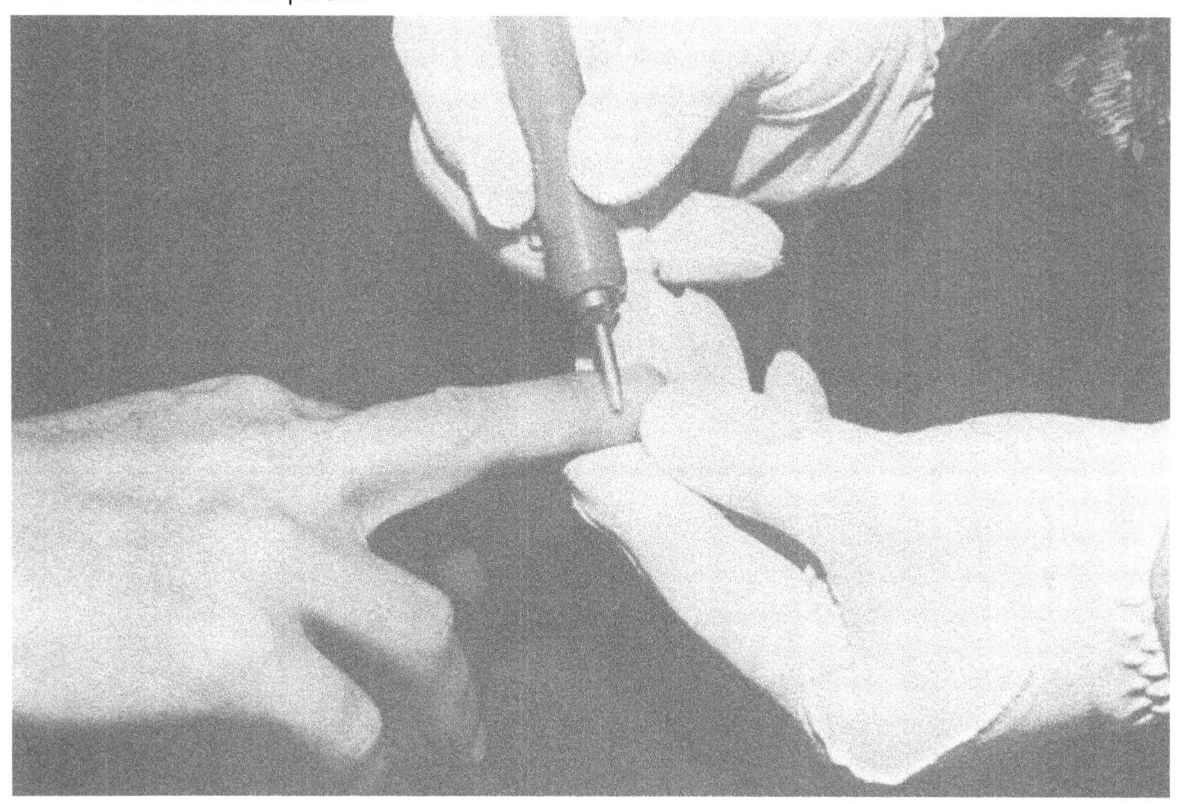

Allergy

2. CMP —Allergy.

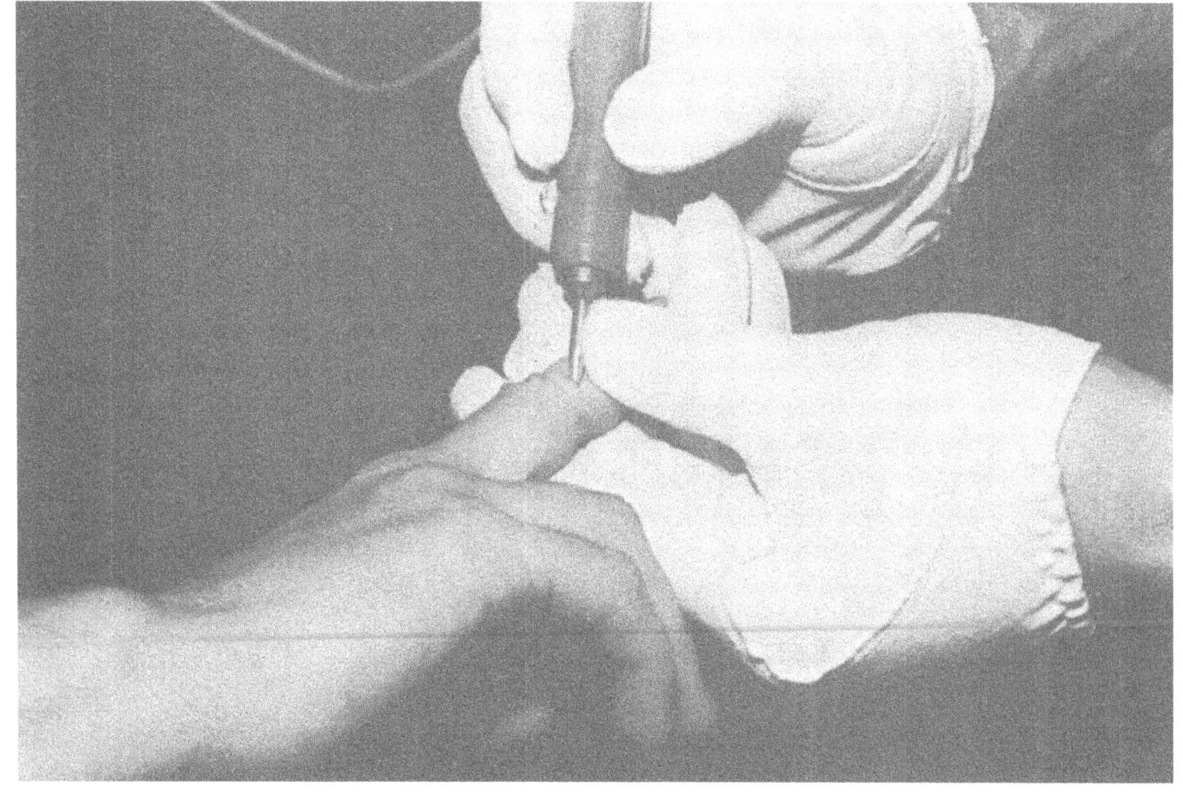

Allergy

3. Vascular sclerosis — Arteriosclerosis.

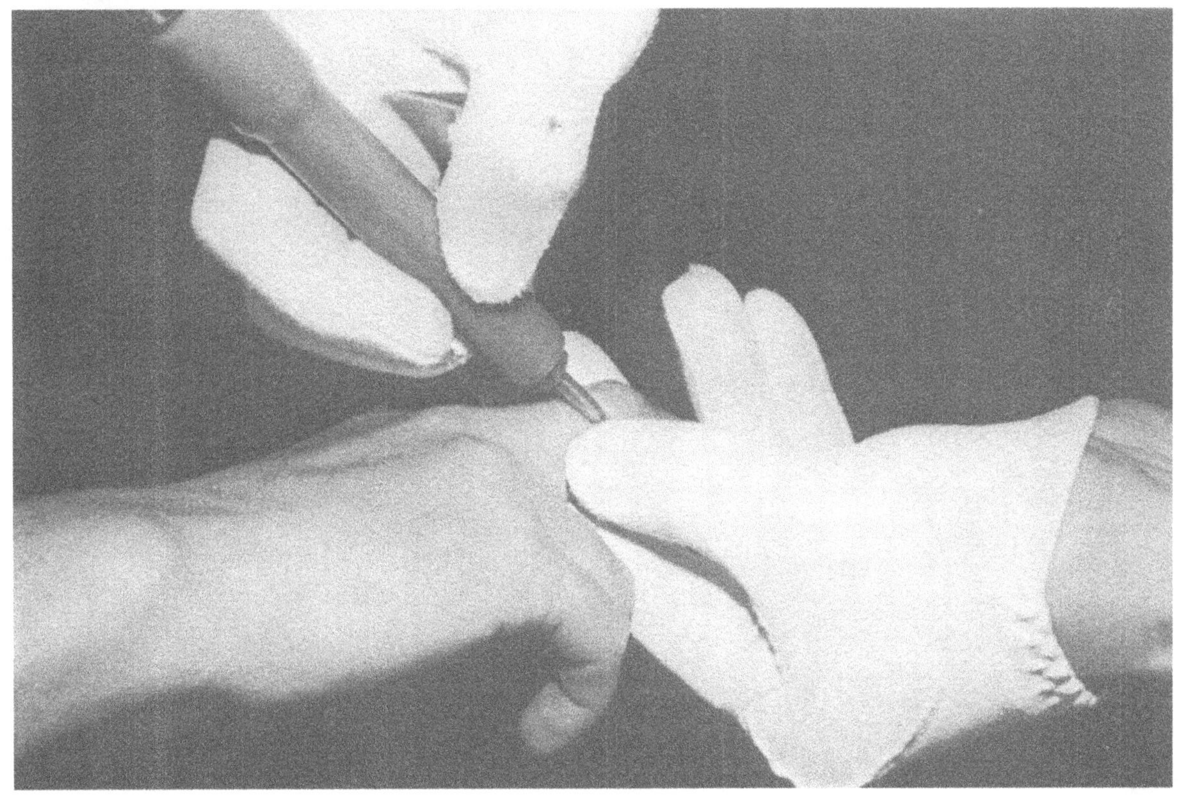

Allergy

4. MP-2 — Skin of upper portion of the body.

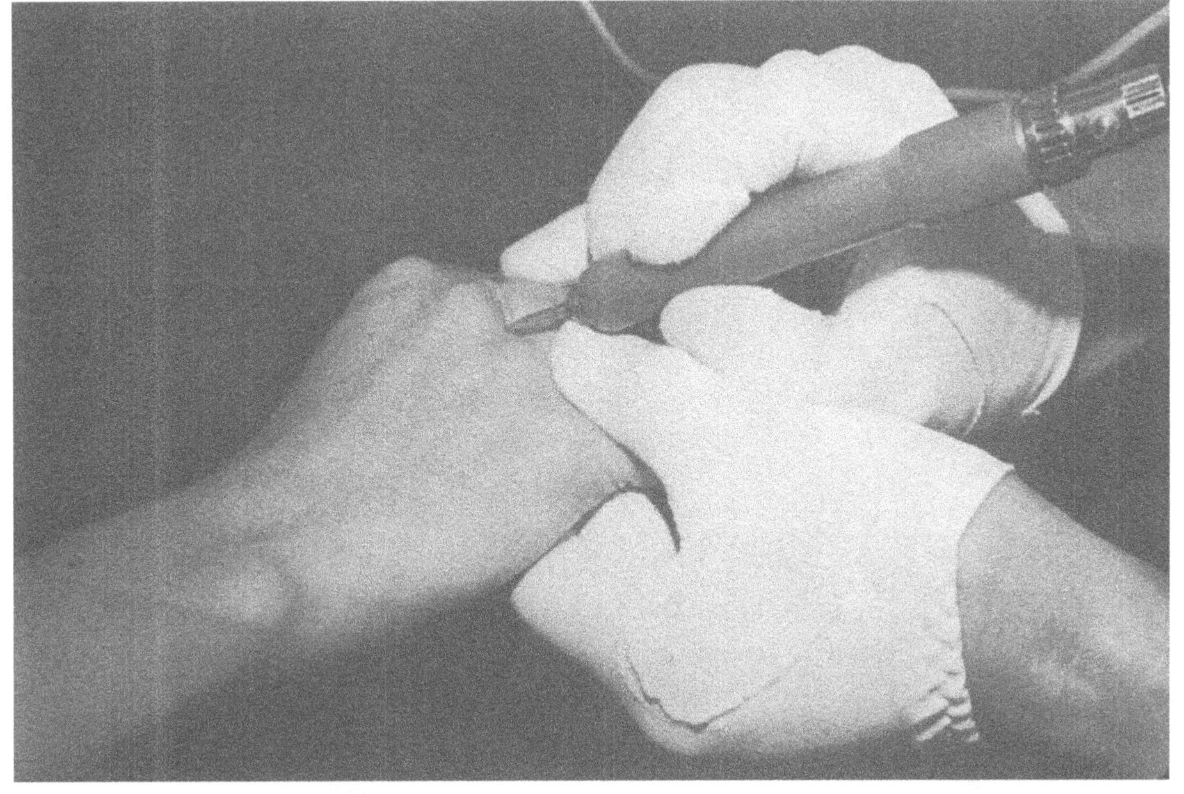

Allergy

5. MP-3 — Skin of the head, allergies of organs of the head, oral cavity, nasal and paranasal sinus.

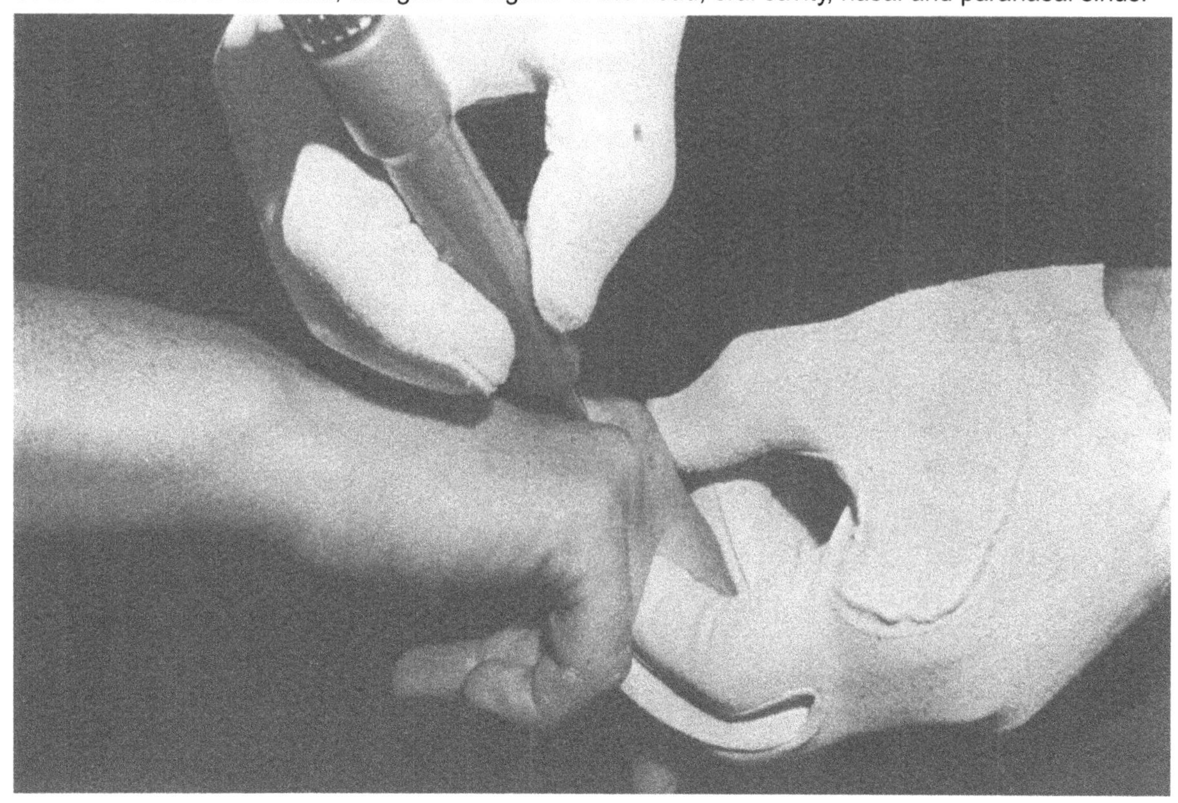

NOTES

Organ Degeneration (parenchymal or epithelial degeneration)

Voll's *Illustrated Volume II,* fig. 31, p. 71.

1. MP-1 — Organs of abdomen, pelvis, Li.
2. CMP — Organ degeneration of entire body.
3. MP Entire — peritoneum — both for cancer.
4. MP Entire — pleura — both for cancer (Hodgkin's Disease), distal middle knuckle.
5. MP-2 — Organs in chest and neck.
6. MP-3 — Organs in head (after stroke, compare with nerve degeneration MP-3).
7. MP-4 — Organs in abdomen and pelvis.

NOTES

Organ Degeneration

1. MP-1 — Organs of abdomen, pelvis, Li.

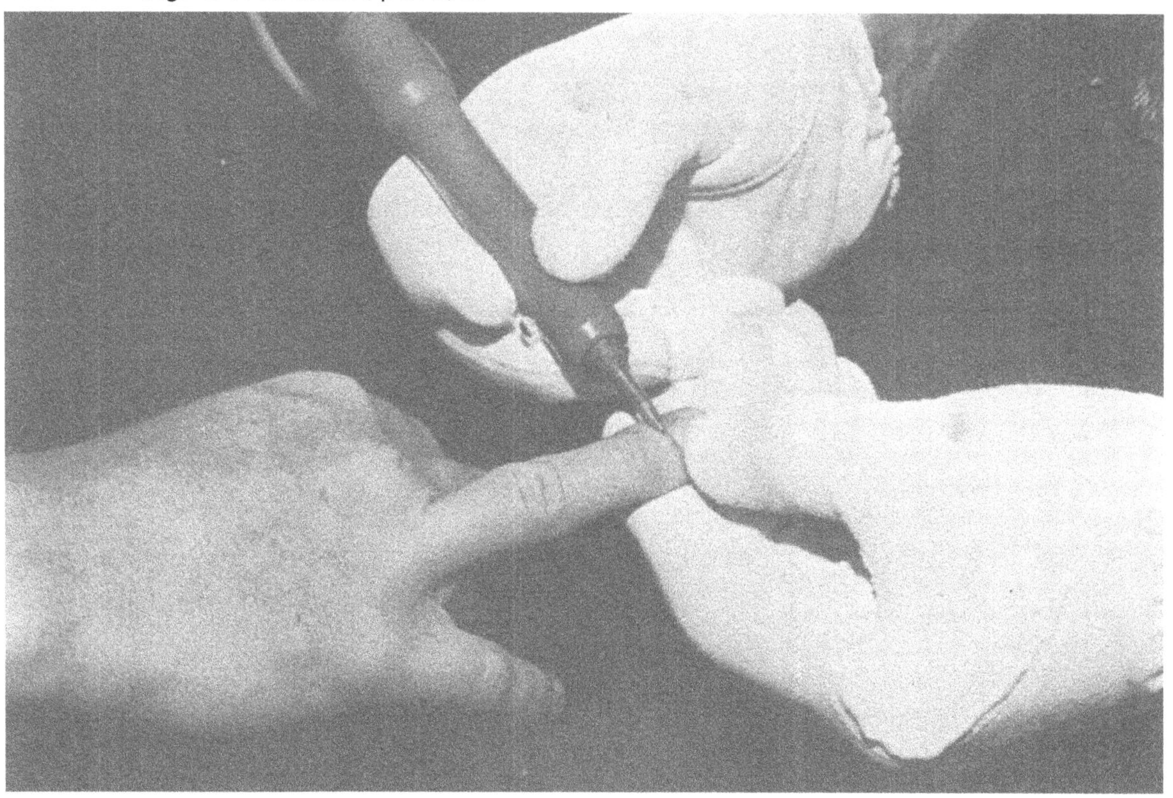

Organ Degeneration

2. CMP — Organ degeneration of entire body.

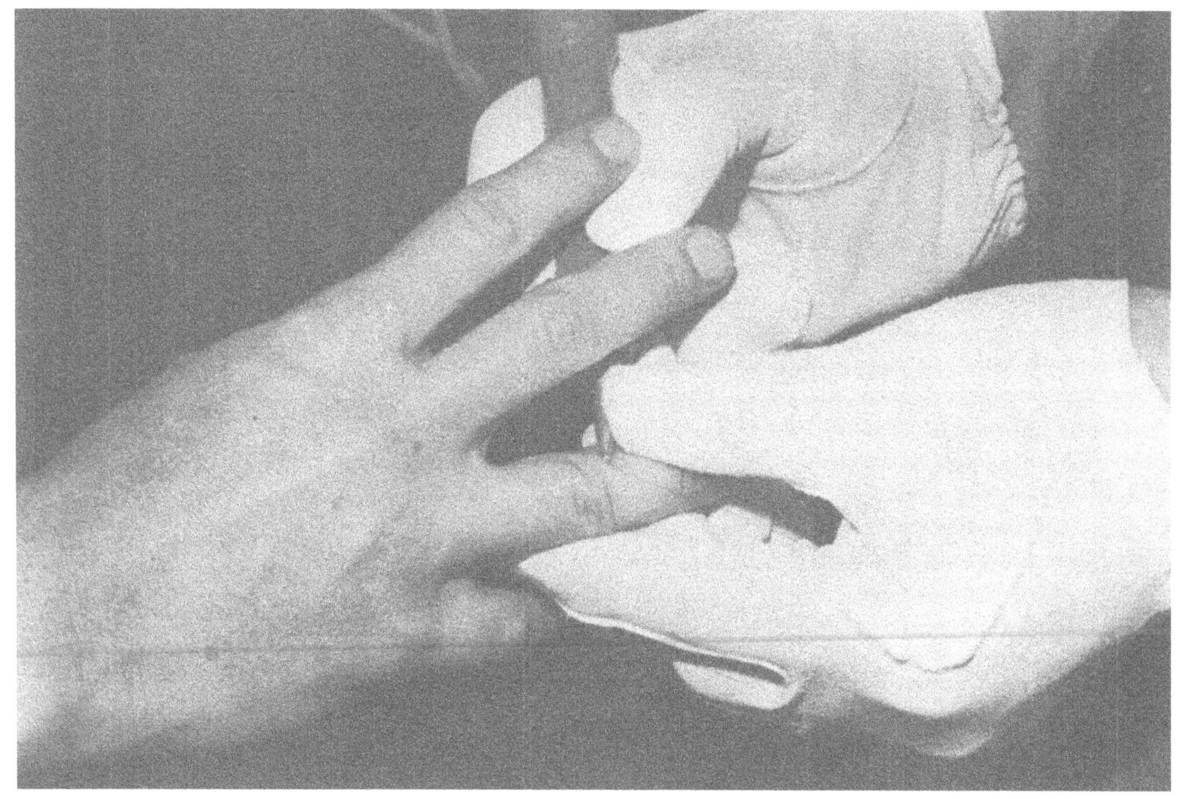

Organ Degeneration

3. MP Entire — peritoneum — both for cancer.

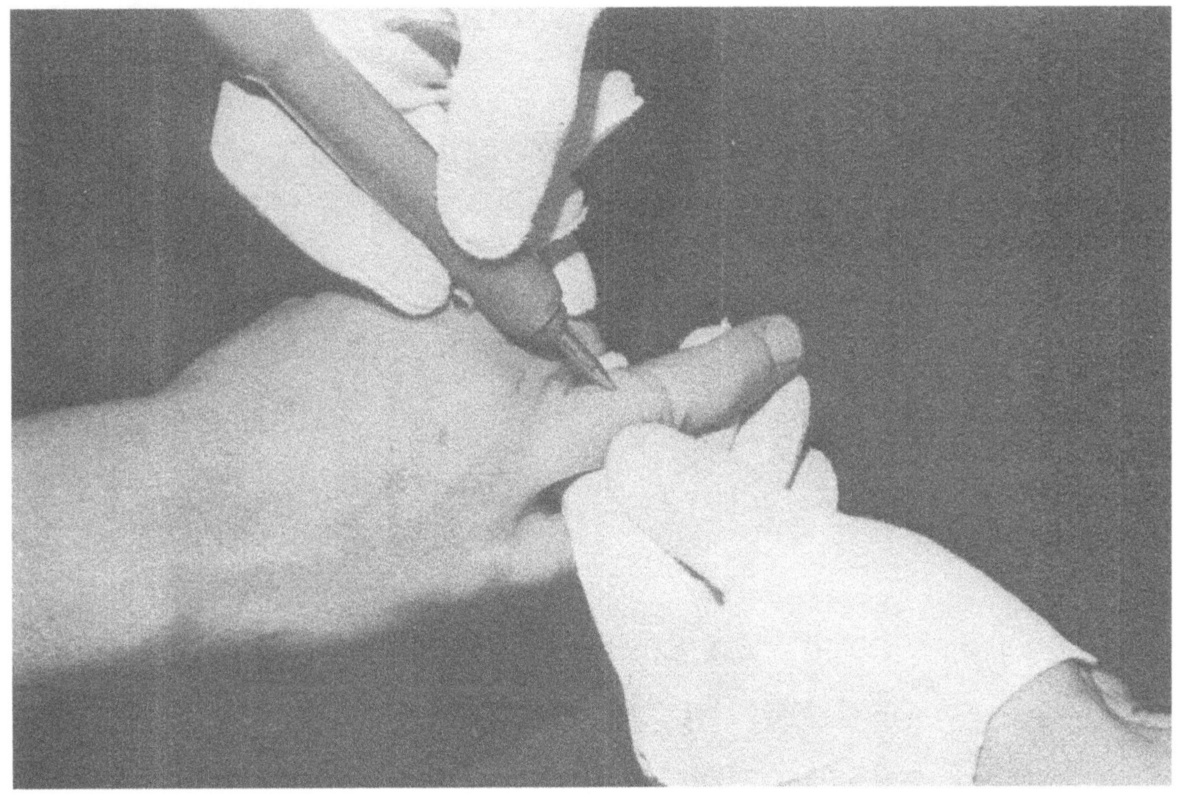

Organ Degeneration

4. MP Entire — pleura — both for cancer (Hodgkin's Disease), distal middle knuckle.

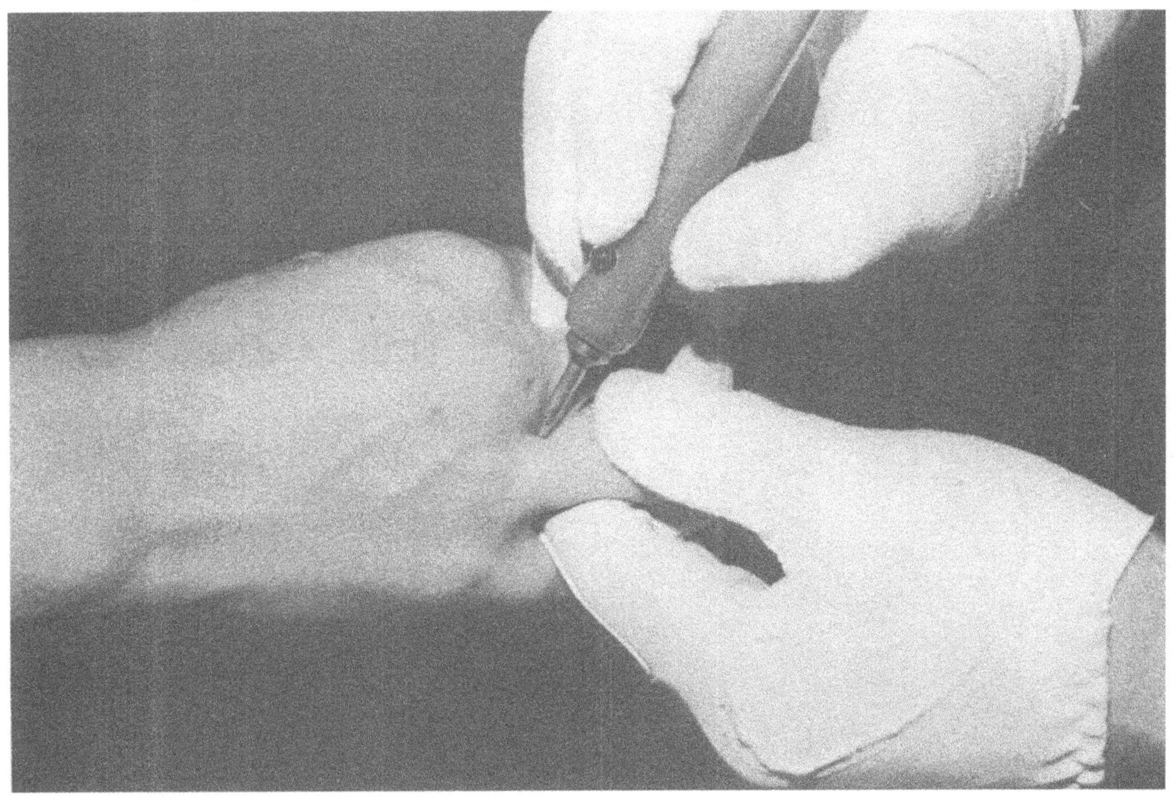

Organ Degeneration

5. MP-2 — Organs in chest and neck.

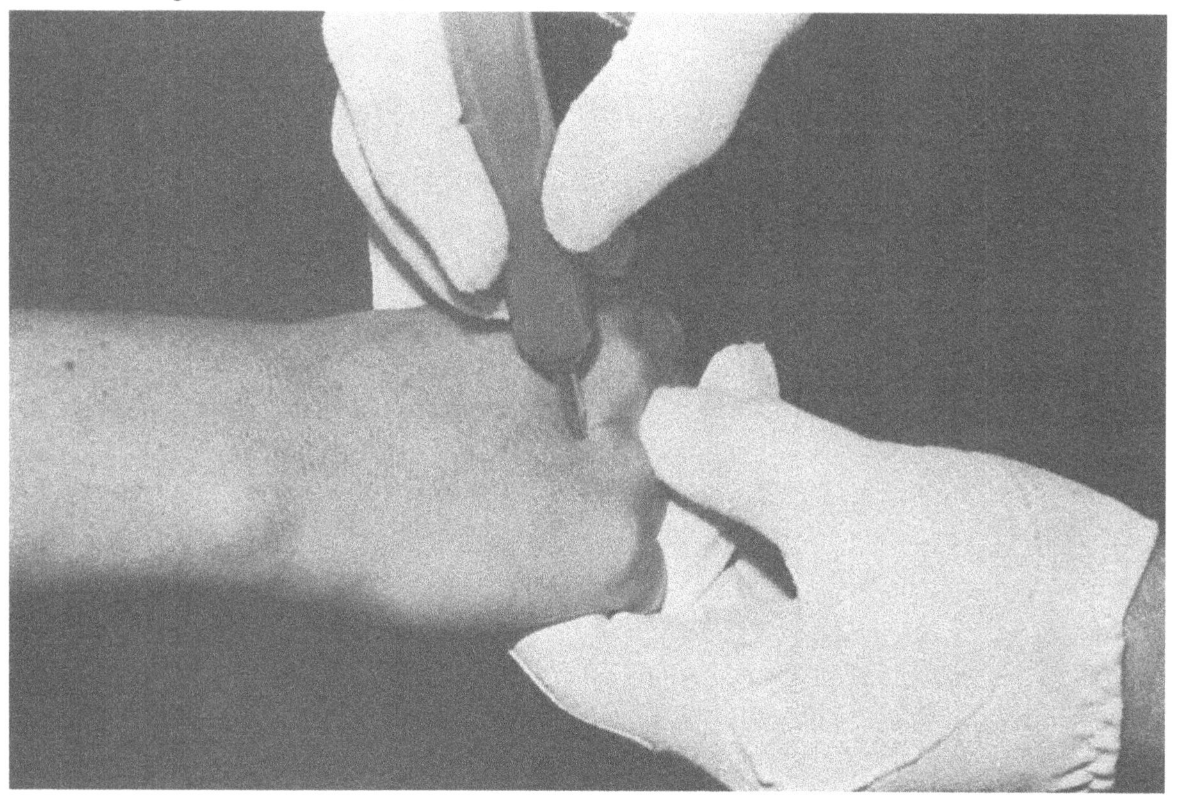

Organ Degeneration

6. MP-3 — Organs in head (after stroke, compare with nerve degeneration MP-3).

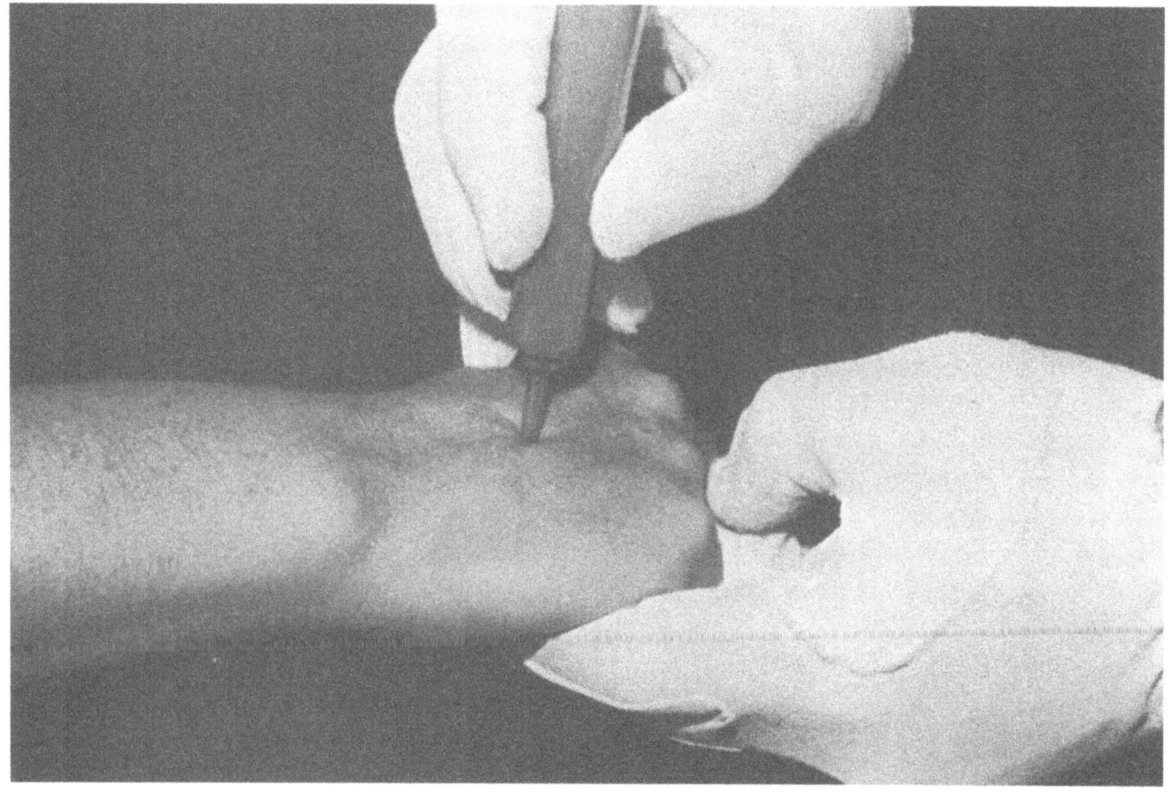

Endocrine (T.W.)

Voll's *Illustrated Volume II, fig. 23, p. 55.*

1. MP-1 —Adrenal (check Ki-10a, Ki-1 Ob, BL-22, gonad — check BL-65: hypoglycemia point — check Ki-1 b).
2. CMP — Endocrine glands.
3. MP — Endocrine pancreas function (head of pancreas right, tail of pancreas left).
4. MP — Mammary gland (in case of ID on CMP — check St-MP-41 a, organ degeneration MP-2, fibroid degeneration MP-2, parenchymal and epithelial degeneration MP-2), retromolar pad system.
5. MP-TW-2 — Summation for thyroid St-10, parathyroid St-9 (mineral metabolism), thymus St-11 (check for cancer).
6. MP-TW-3 —Pineal gland BL-8; pituitary gland: anterior lobe GBL-21, SI-15, TW-16; intermediate lobe GBL-20a, posterior lobe GBL-12.
7. MP-TW-16a — Deep cervical lymph nodes.
   a. MP-Tonsillar ring of 5 tonsils.
   b. MP-Lymph 2 — Dental, upper and lower jaw.
   c. MP-Lymph 3 — Paranasal sinus.
   d. MP-TW-1a — Cervical part of the sympathetic nerve.
   e. MP-Circulation 8e — Left thoracic aorta and thoracic aortic plexus. aorta plexus.
   f. MP-Circulation 9 — Arteries.
   g. MP-Lymph 1 — Palatine tonsil.
8. MP-TW-17 — Middle Ear.
9. MP-TW-18 — Internal ear.
10. MP-TW-20 — Hypothalamus (above ear) for vegetative functions.

Endocrine

1. MP-1 — Adrenal.

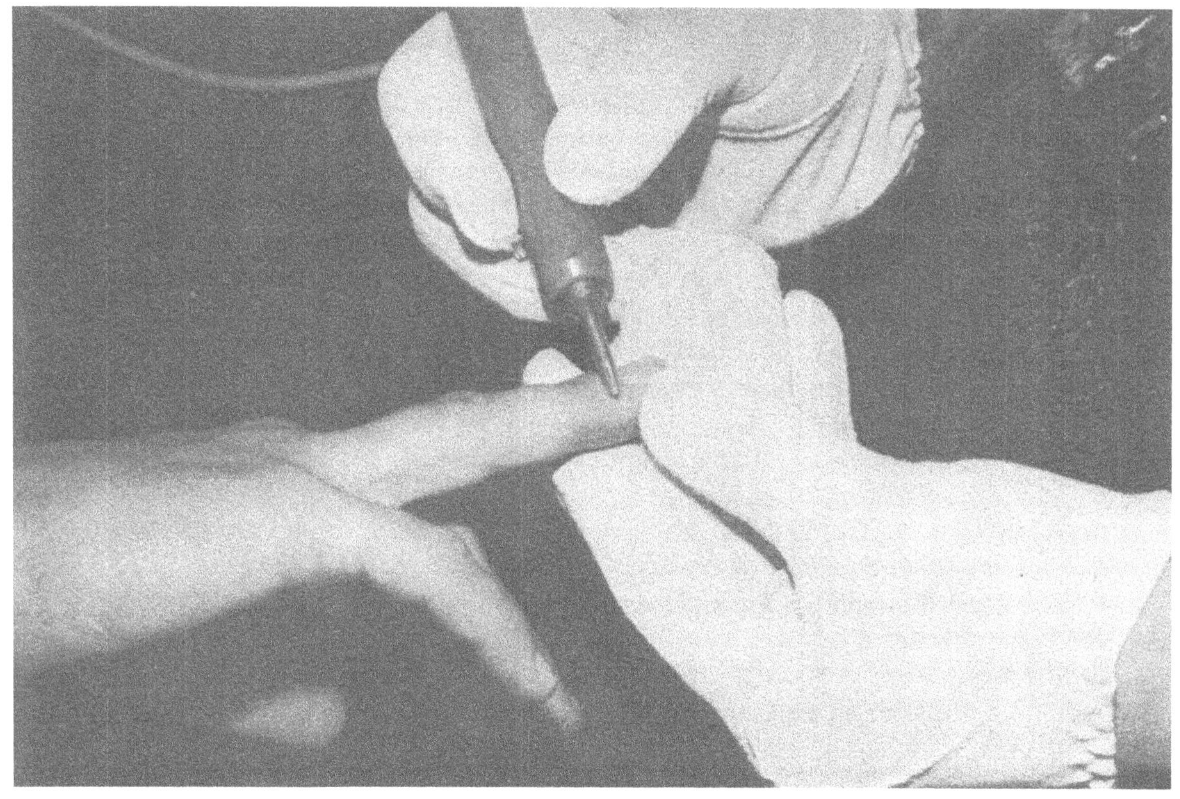

Endocrine

2. CMP — Endocrine glands.

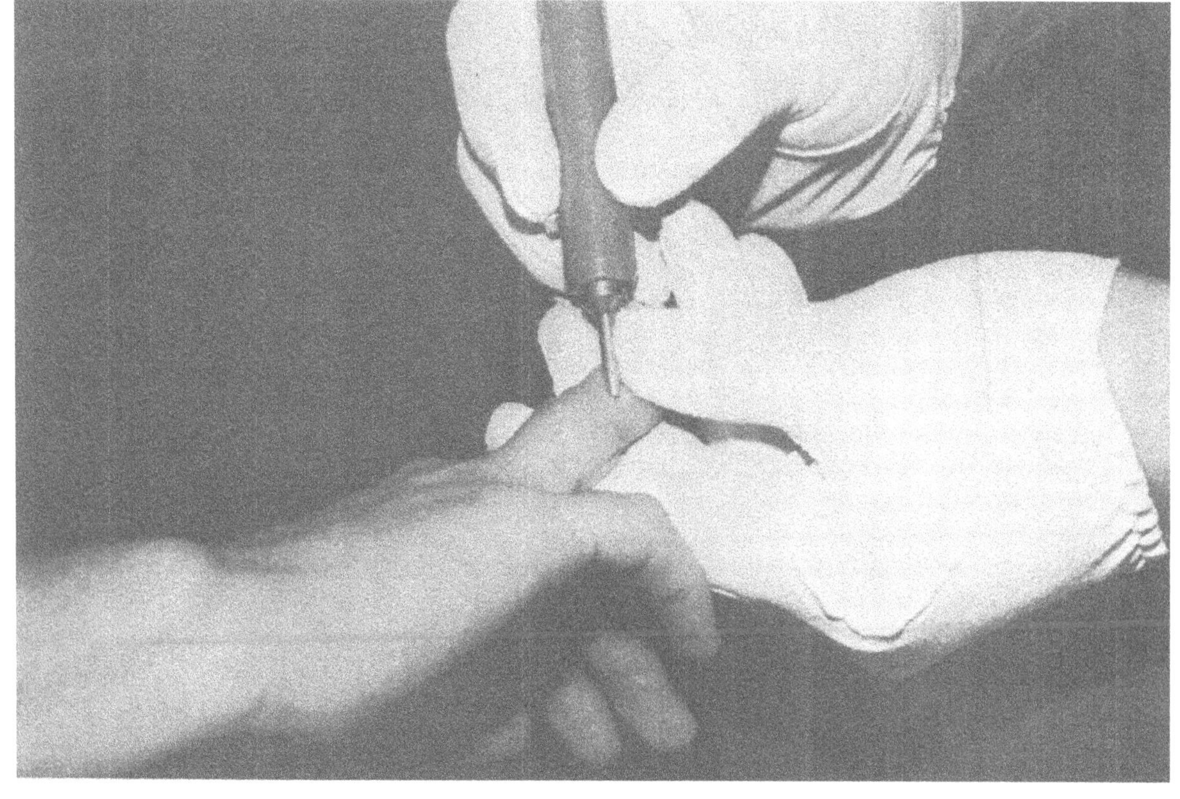

Endocrine

3. MP — Endocrine pancreas function.

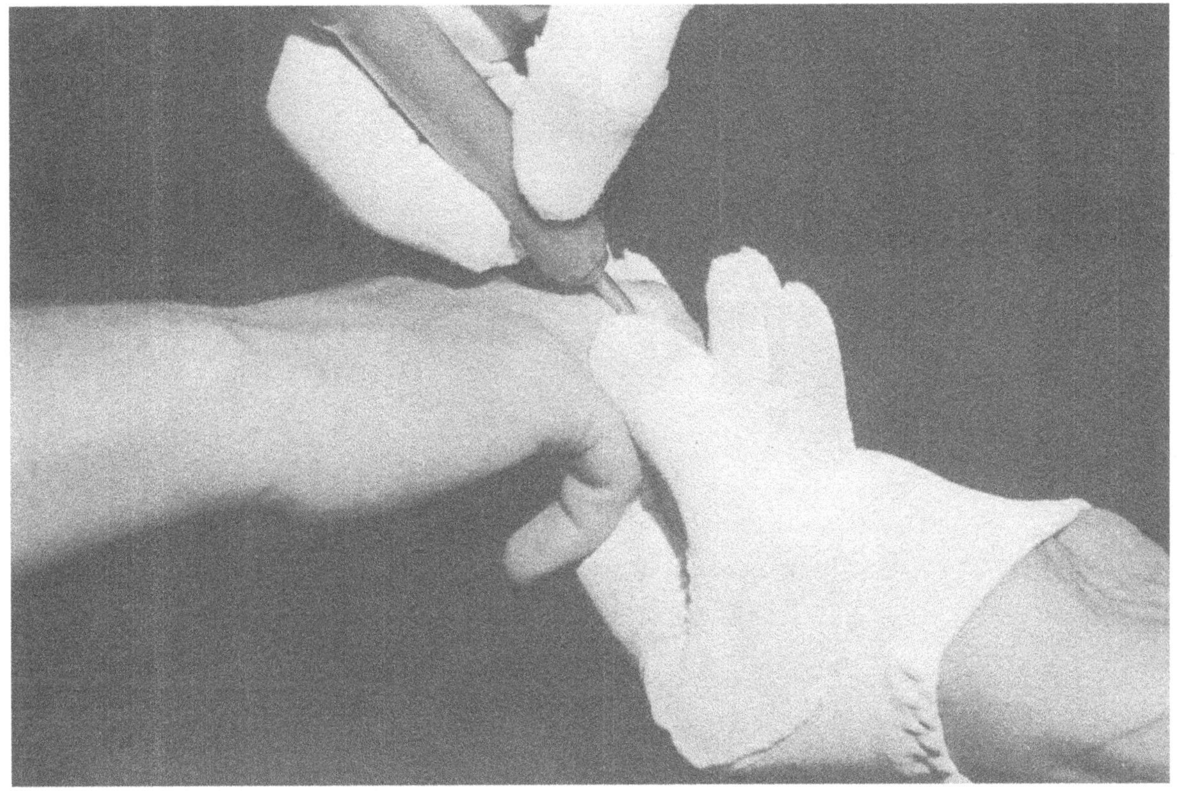

Endocrine

4. MP — Mammary gland.

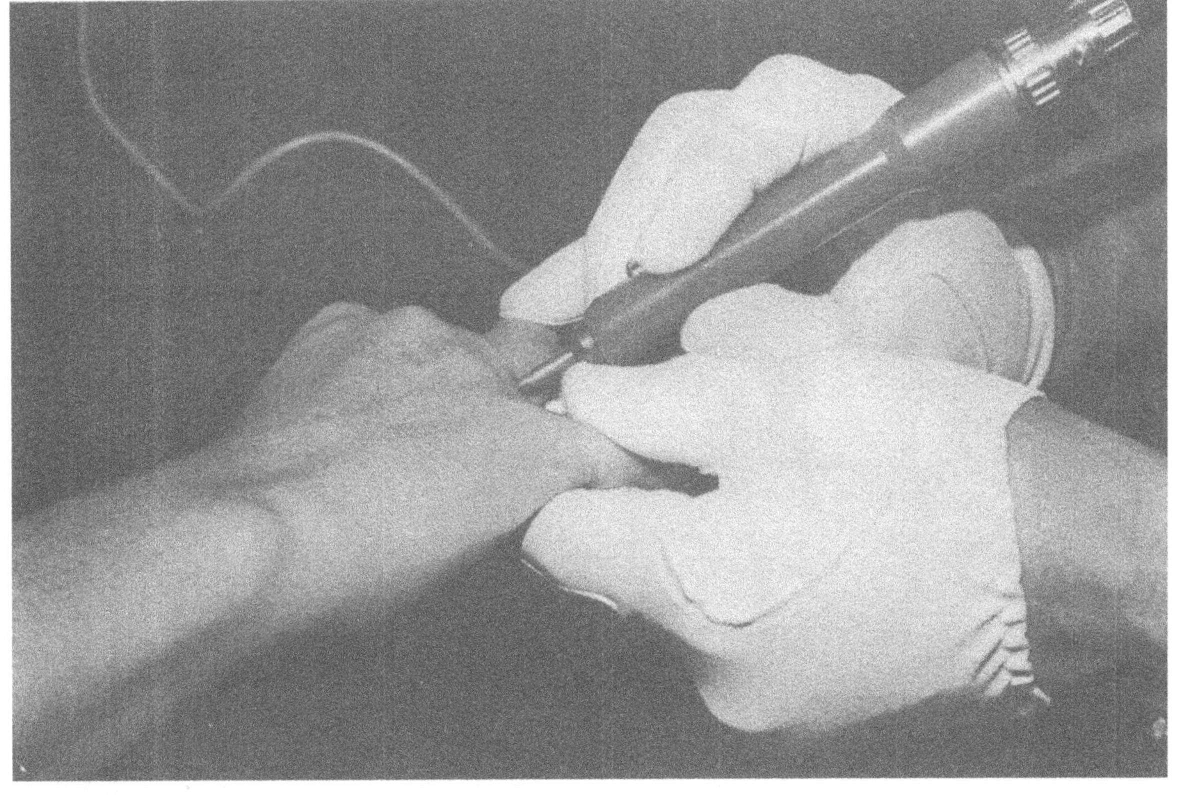

Endocrine

5. MP-TW-2 — Summation for thyroid St-10, parathyroid St-9 (mineral metabolism), thymus St-11.

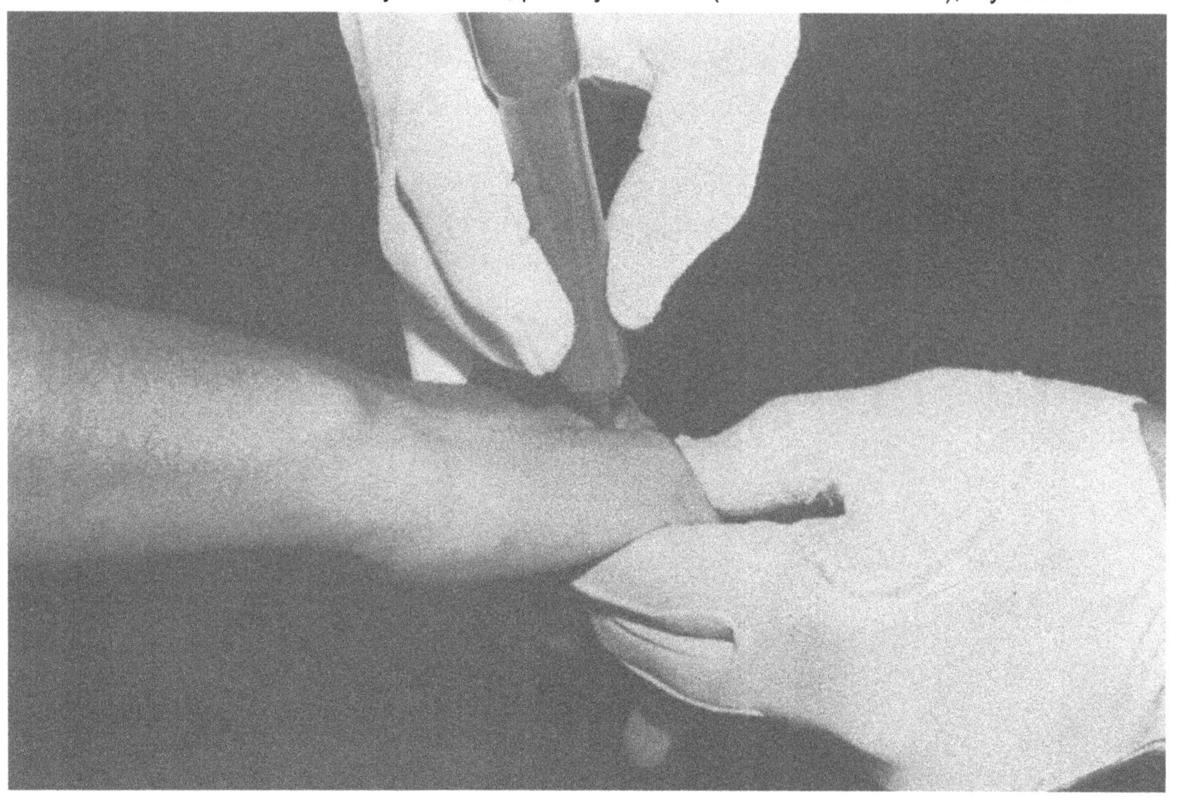

Endocrine

6. MP-TW-3 — Pineal gland BL-8; pituitary gland.

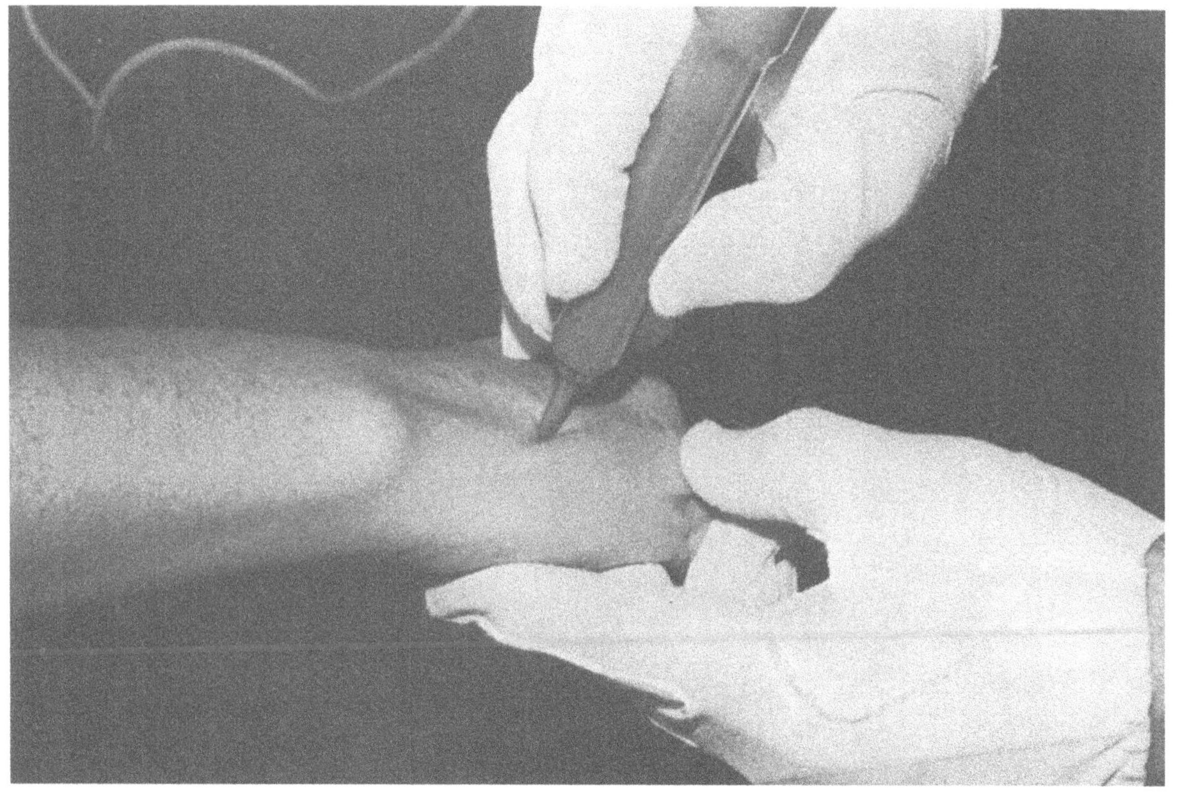

Heart

Voll's *Illustrated Volume II,* fig. 1a, p. 10; fig. 1b, p. 11.

RIGHT

1. MP-9 — Pulmonary valve (pneumonia).
2. CMP —Heart.
3. MP-8a — Pericardium.
4. MP-8 — Tricuspid valve (palm side).
5. *MP-7 — Conduction System.*
6. MP-6 — Cardiac muscle.

LEFT

1. MP-9 — Aortic valve.
2. CMP —Heart.
3. MP-8a — Pericardium.
4. MP-8 — Mitrial valve (palm side).
5. MP-7 — Conduction System.
6. MP-6 — Cardiac muscle.

NOTES

Heart

1. MP-9 — Pulmonary valve (pneumonia), right. 1. MP-9 — Aortic valve, left.

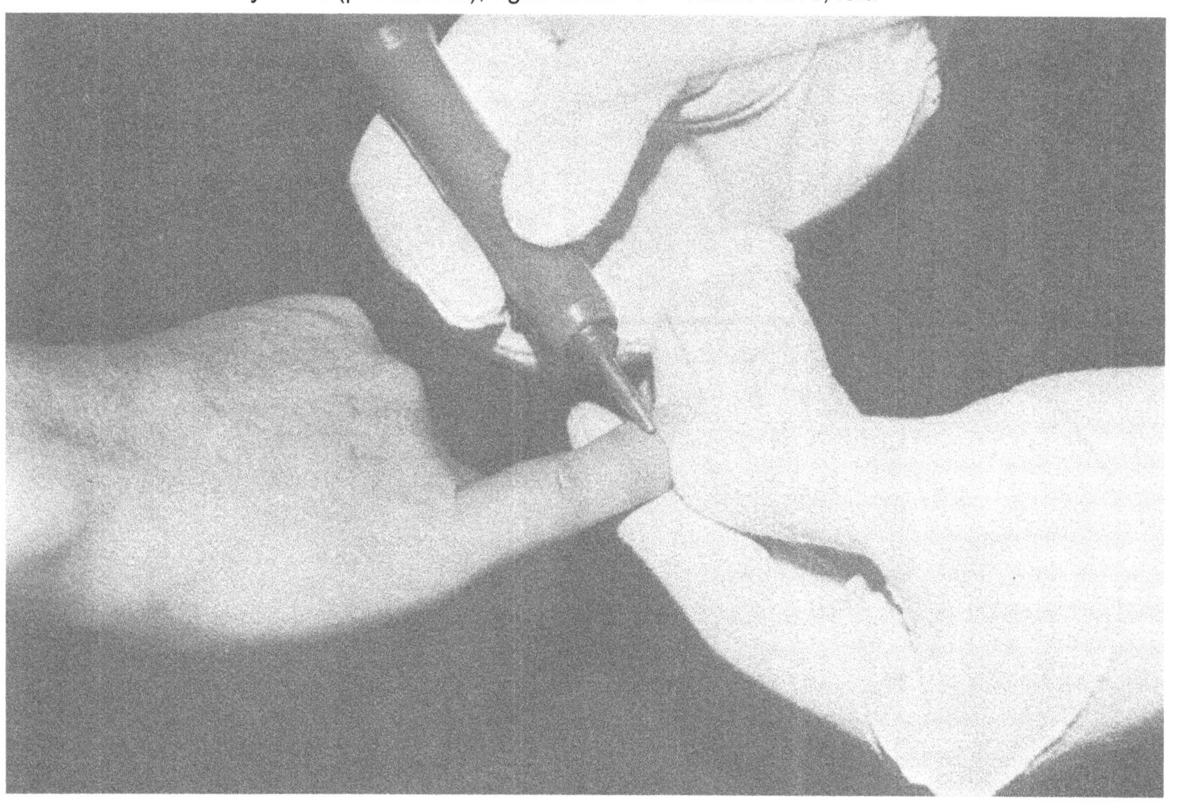

Heart

2. CMP —Heart, right. 2. CMP — Heart, left.

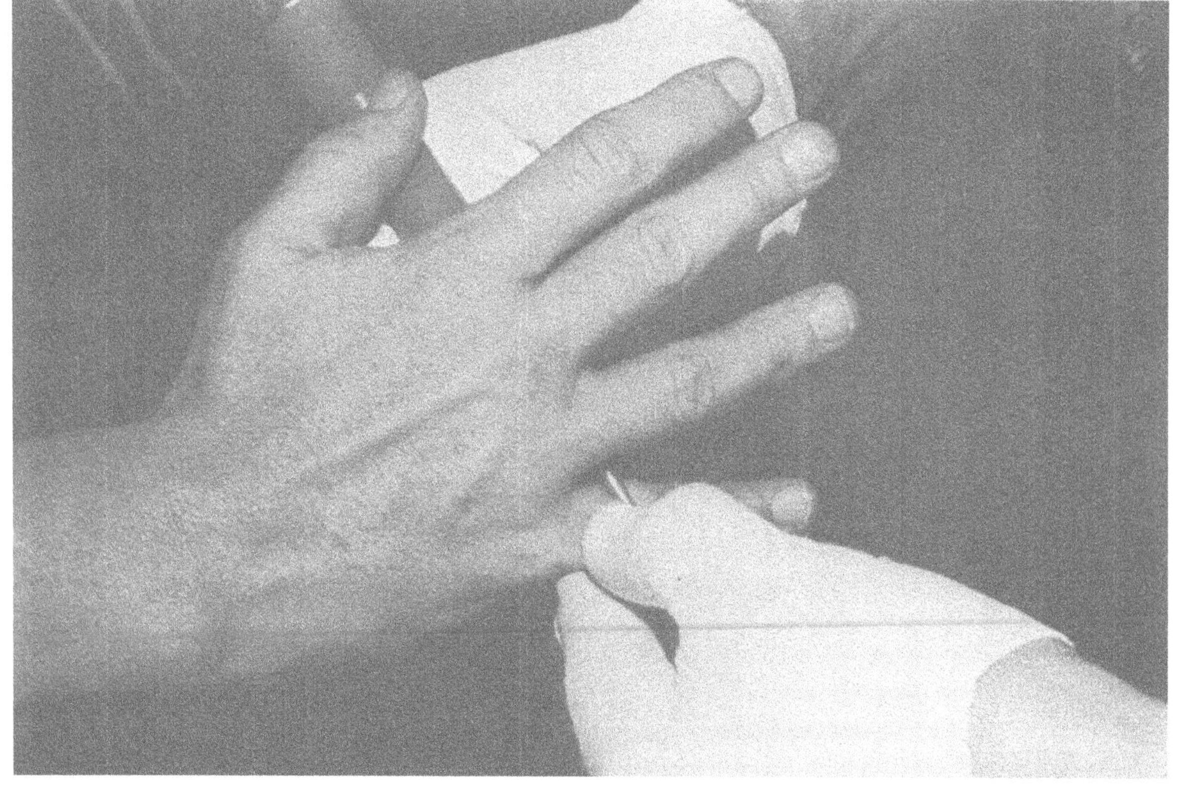

Heart

3. MP-8a— Pericardium, right. 3. MP-8a — Pericardium, left.

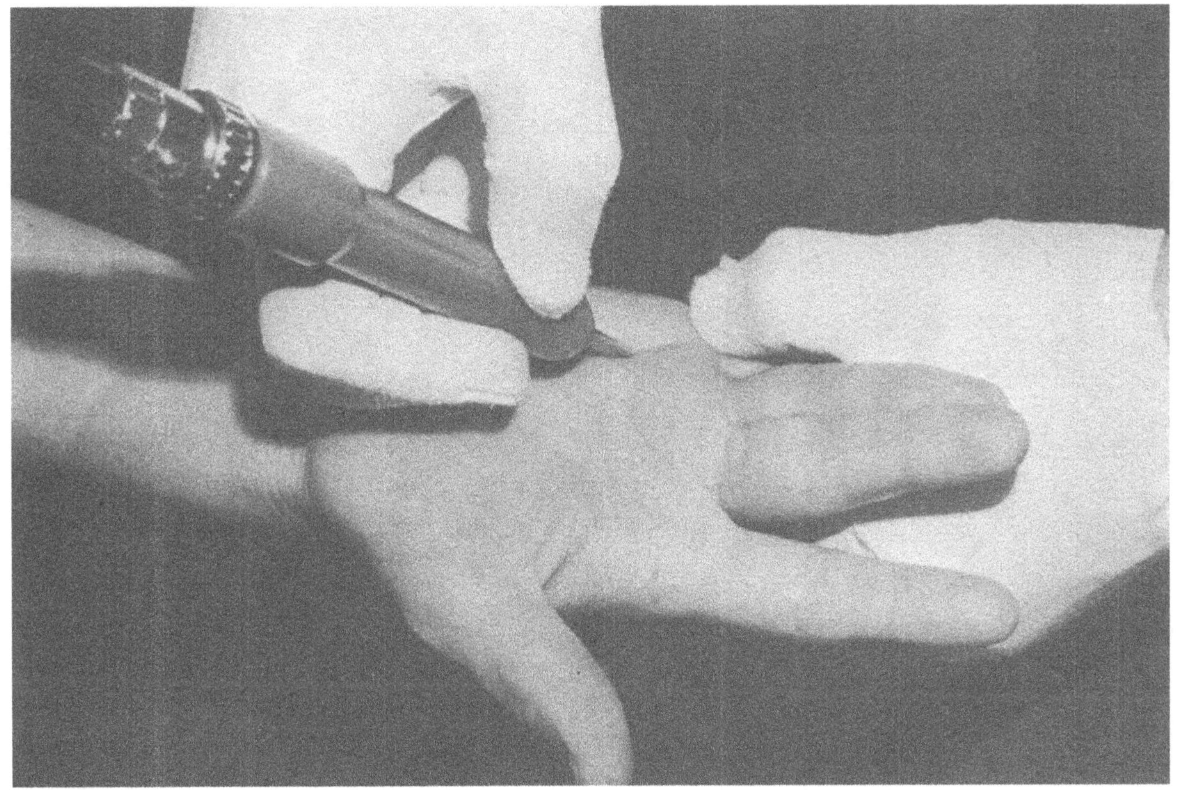

Heart

4. MP-8 — Tricuspid valve (palm side), right 4. MP-8 — Mitrial valve (palm side), left.

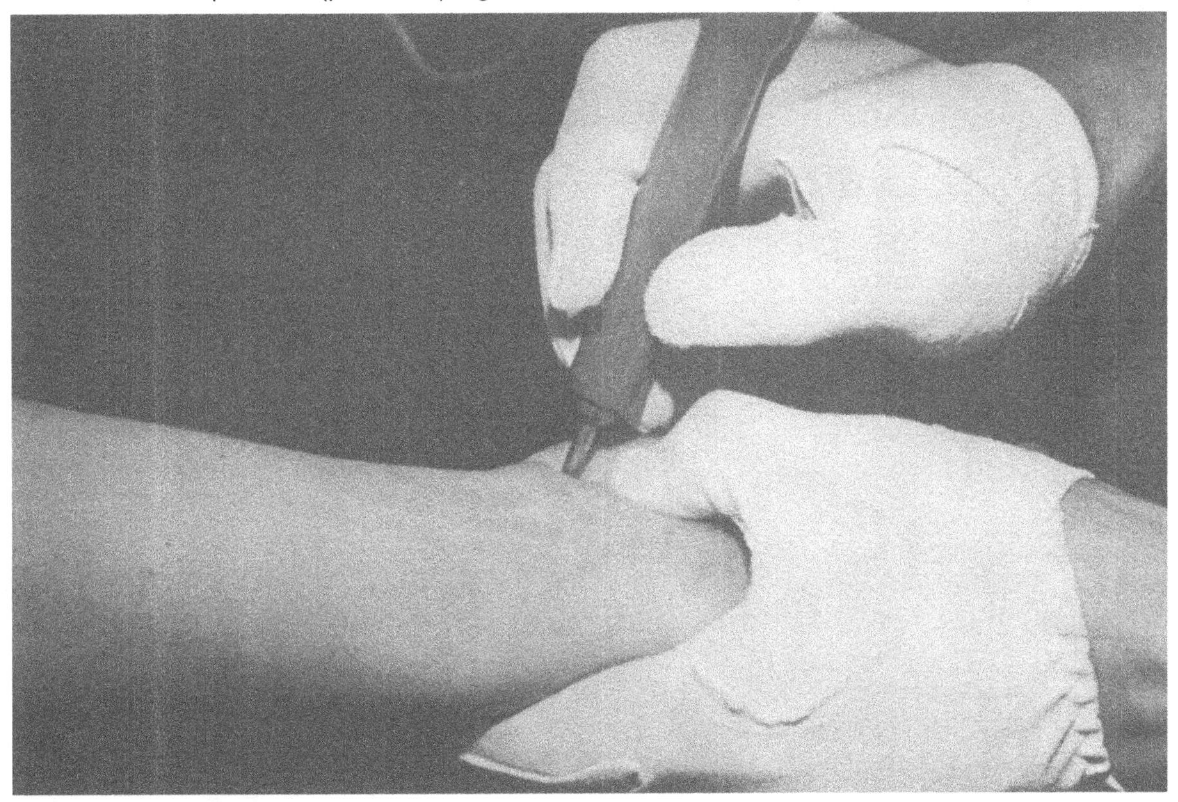

Heart

6. MP-6 — Cardiac muscle, right. 6. MP-6 — Cardiac muscle, left.

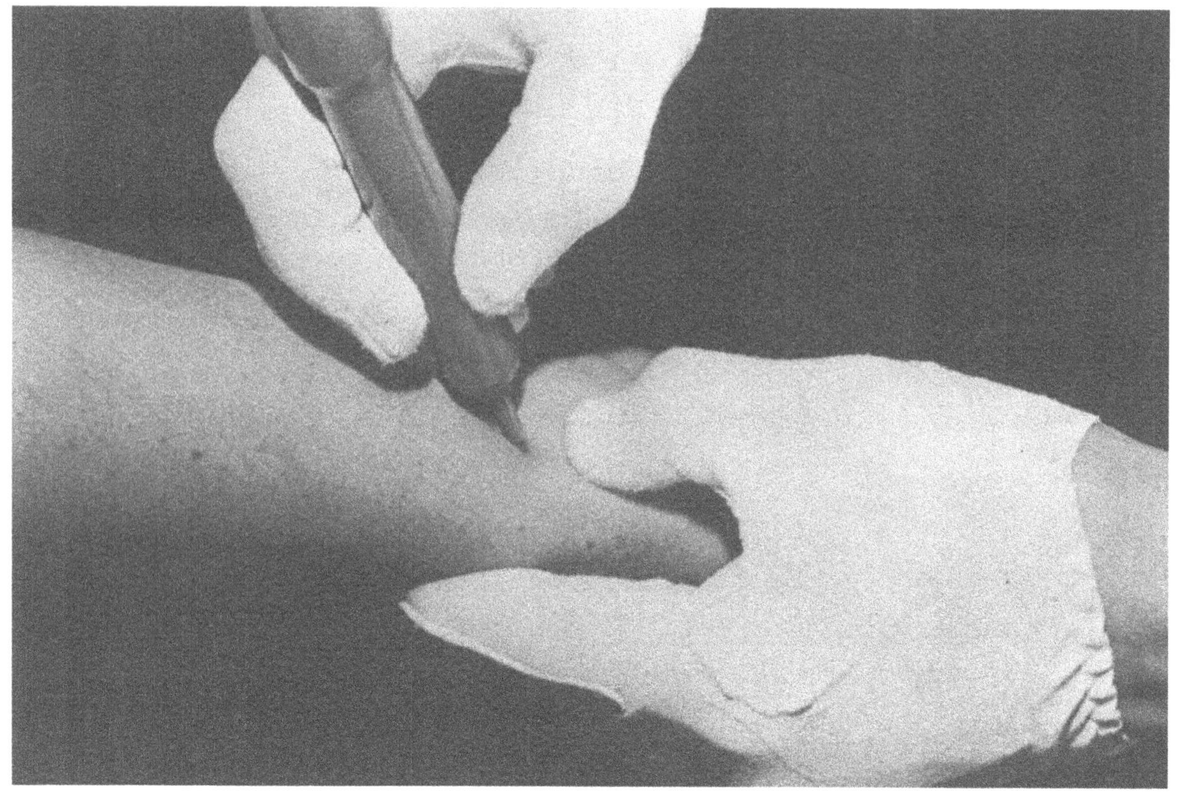

NOTES

Small Intestine

Voll's *Illustrated Volume II*, fig. 10a, p. 28.
Illness of the SI may affect the brain, heart, ear and central and peripheral nervous system.

RIGHT

1. MP-1 — Ileum, terminal portion ileo-cecal valve. Both sides (tennis elbow measurement, ear ringings). Pain at 1-3 p.m. in lower right abdomen from the terminal ileum. Indication is the ileitis terminalis (Crohn Disease).
2. MP-1a — Upper mesenteric plexus.
3. CMP — Whole SI.
4. MP — Peritoneum.
5. MP-2 — Duodenum, lower horizontal portion.
6. MP-3 — Duodenum, descending portion both sides (ulcer duodenum — general tiredness because the brain does not have enough food). Also check for normalization of the nerve degeneration CMP because of the lack of food to the nerve degeneration.
7. MP-4 — Horizontal upper portion of duodenum.
8. *MP-6 — Cervical, spine, neck.*
9. *MP-7 — Nerves for upper extremity (if ID on nerve degeneration* MP-2*).*
10. *MP-8 — Elbow joints (tennis elbow).*
11. *MP-9 — Muscle of the arm.*

LEFT

1. MP-1 — Ileum (Meckel's Diverticulum). Both sides (tennis elbow measurement, ear ringings).
2. Unknown.
3. CMP — Whole SI.
4. MP — Peritoneum.
5. MP-2 — Jejunum.
6. MP-3 — Flexure between duodenum and jejunum.
7. MP-4 — Ascending portion duodenum (many misdiagnosis of stomach pain).

NOTES

Small Intestine

1. MP-1 — Ileum, terminal portion ileo-cecal valve, right.
1. MP-1 — Ileum (Meckel's Diverticulum), left.

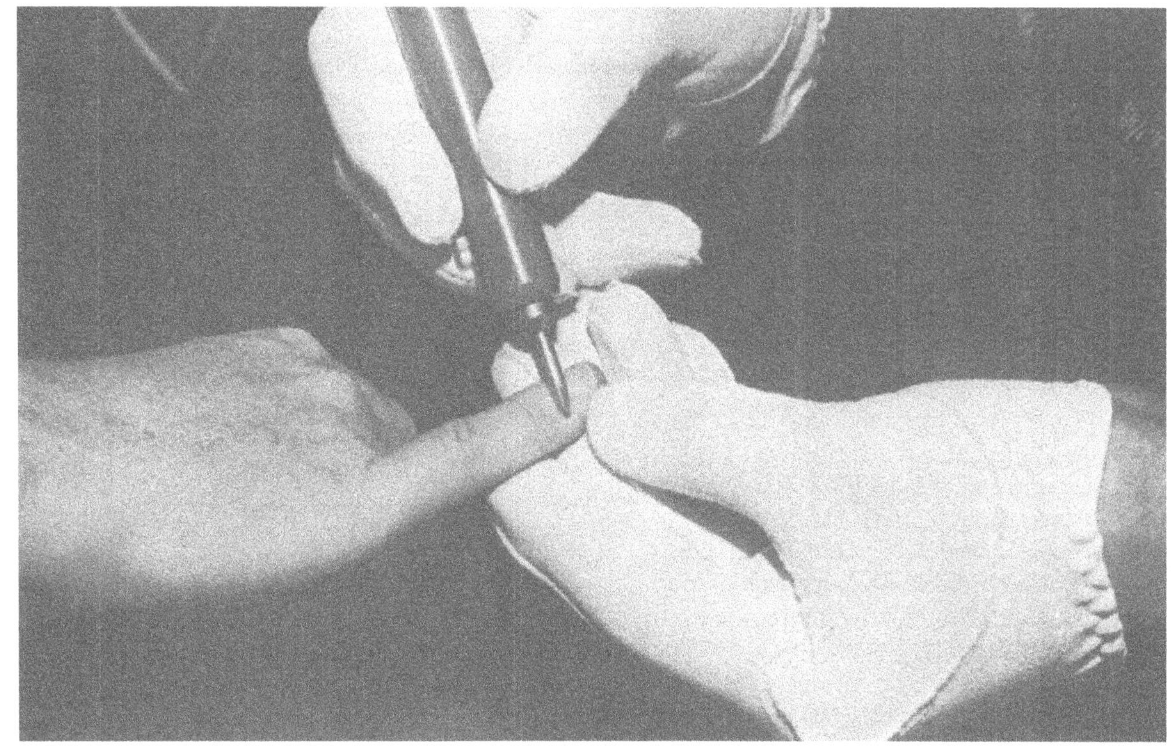

Small Intestine

3. CMP — Whole SI, right. 3. CMP — Whole SI, left.

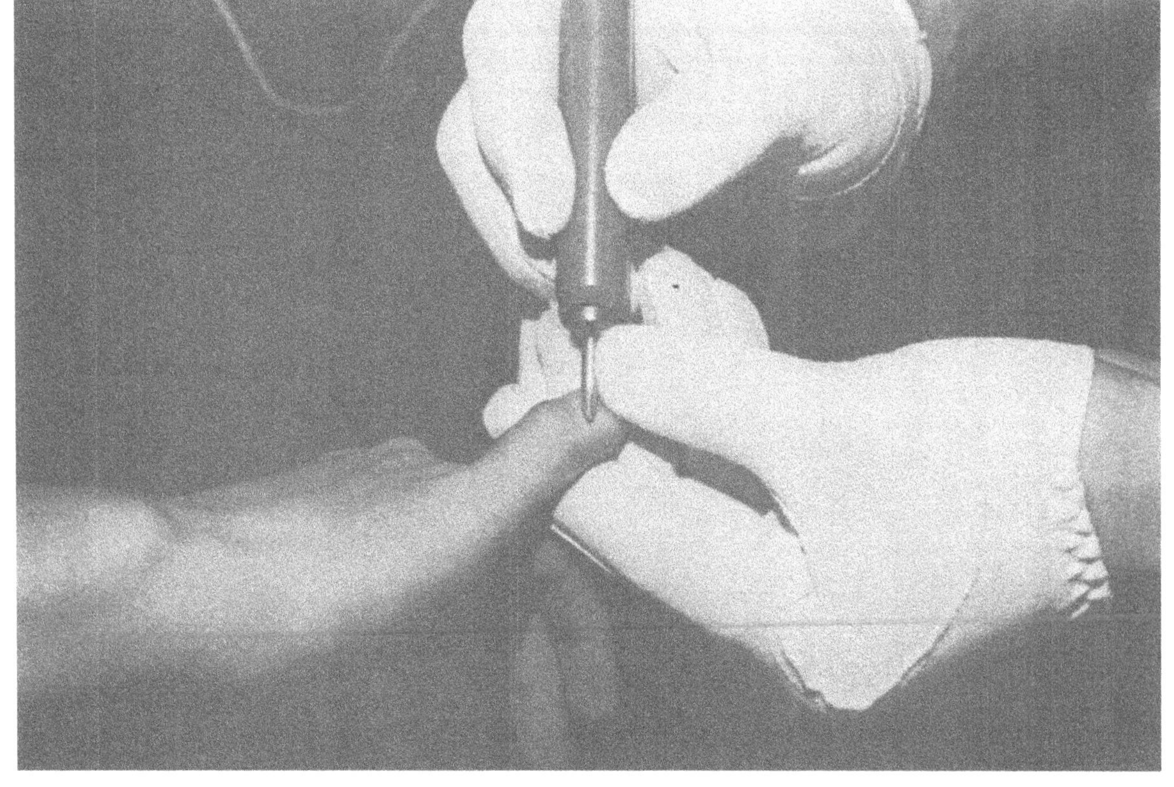

Small Intestine

5. MP-2 — Duodenum, lower horizontal portion, right. 5. MP-2 — Jejunum, left.

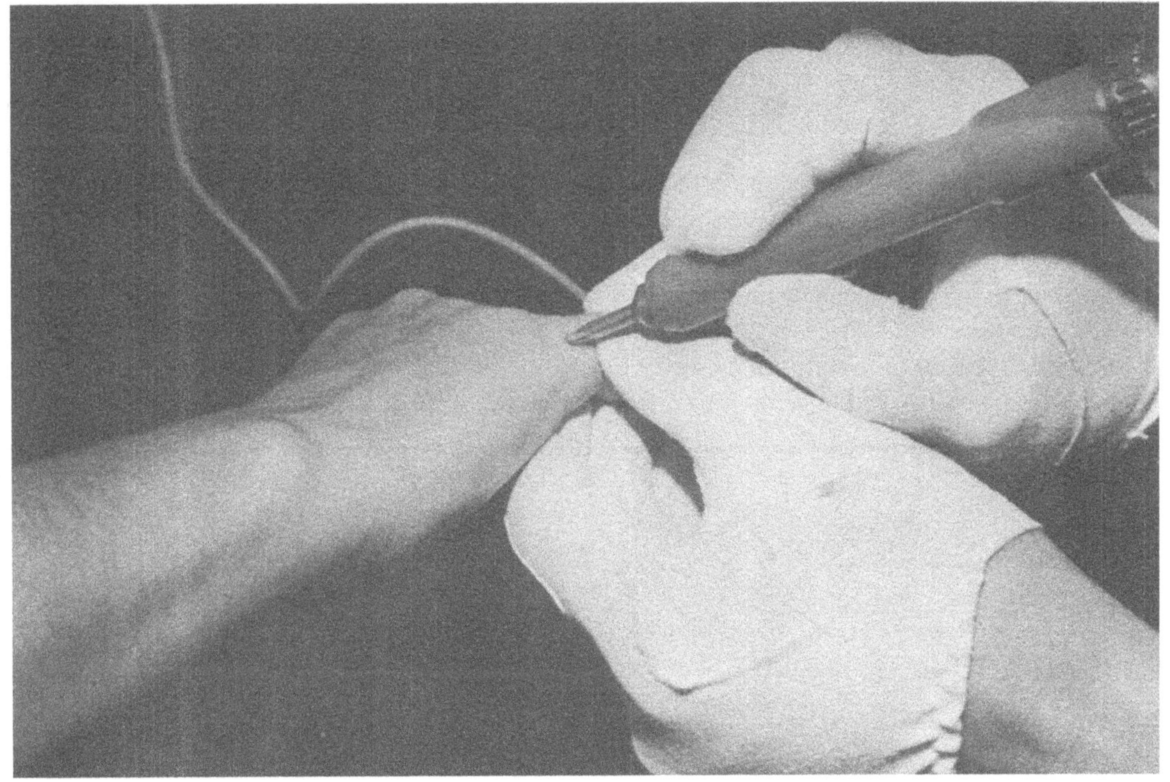

Small Intestine

6. MP-3 — Duodenum, descending portion both sides, right.
6. MP-3 — Flexure between duodenum and jejunum, left.

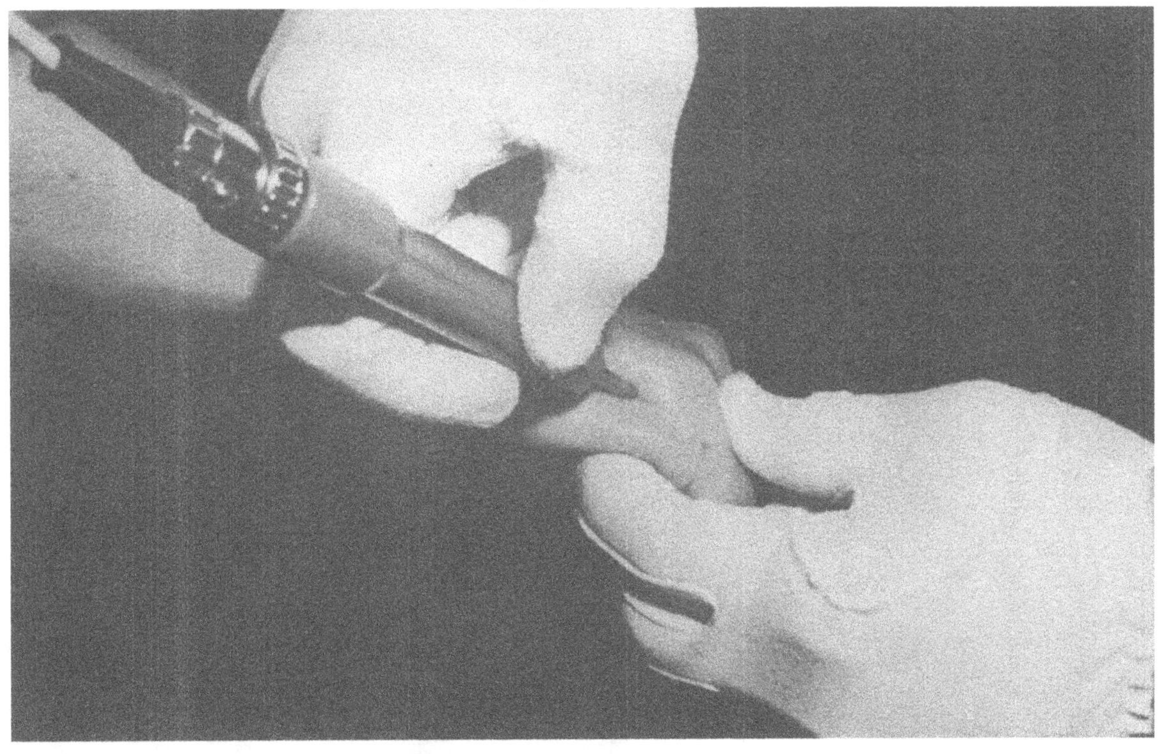

FOOT ELECTRO-ACUPUNCTURE POINTS ACCORDING TO VOLL

Pancreas — Right Side Only

Voll's *Illustrated Volume II*, fig. 11a, p. 30.

1. MP-1 —Protein metabolism.
2. CMP.
3. MP — Peritoneum.
4. MP-2 — Uric acid, high protein diet (disturbance of nucleo-protein metabolism, hyperureimia).
5. MP-3 — CHO point, amylase and maltase (diabetes to 46-44 ID and less than 45, general tiredness of ID).
6. MP-4 — Cholesterol, high lipase, fat metabolism (compare with fat degeneration CMP, hyperlipaemia).
7. *MP-9 — Lymph vessels of lower extremities.*
8. *MP-10 — Venous system of the pelvic region (check for venous congestion).*

NOTES

Pancreas — Right

1. MP-1—Protein metabolism.

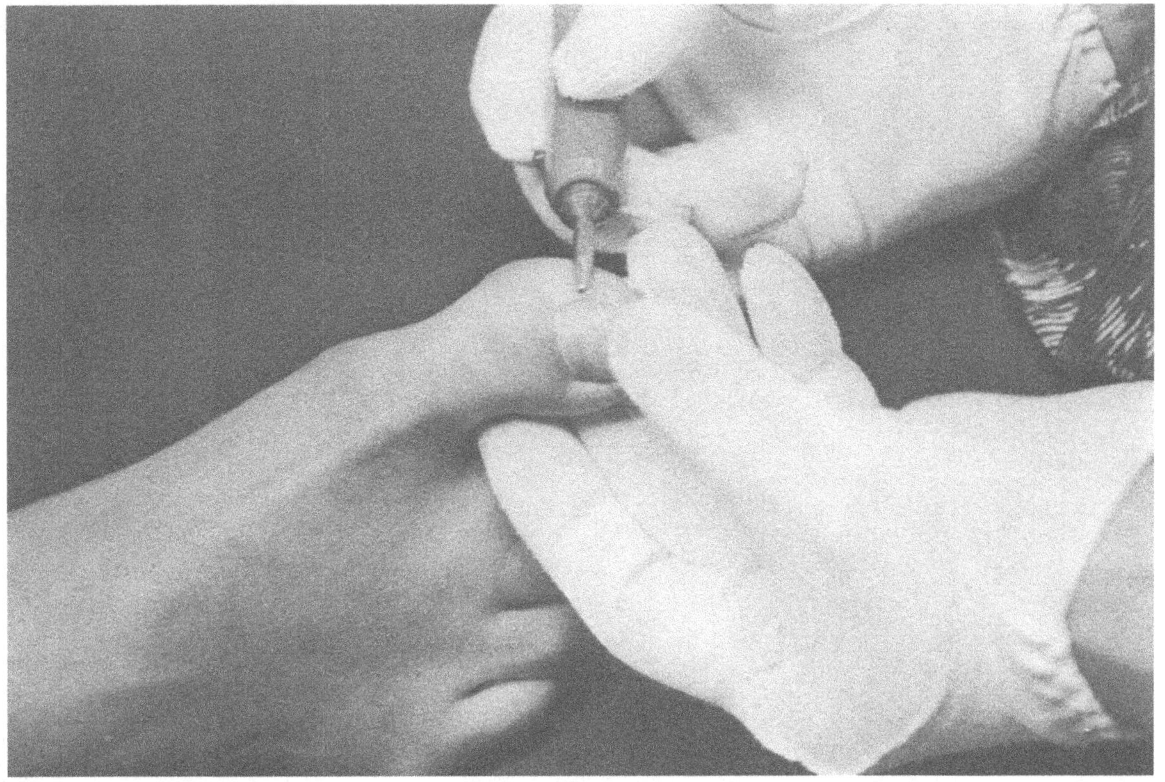

Pancreas — Right

2. CMP.

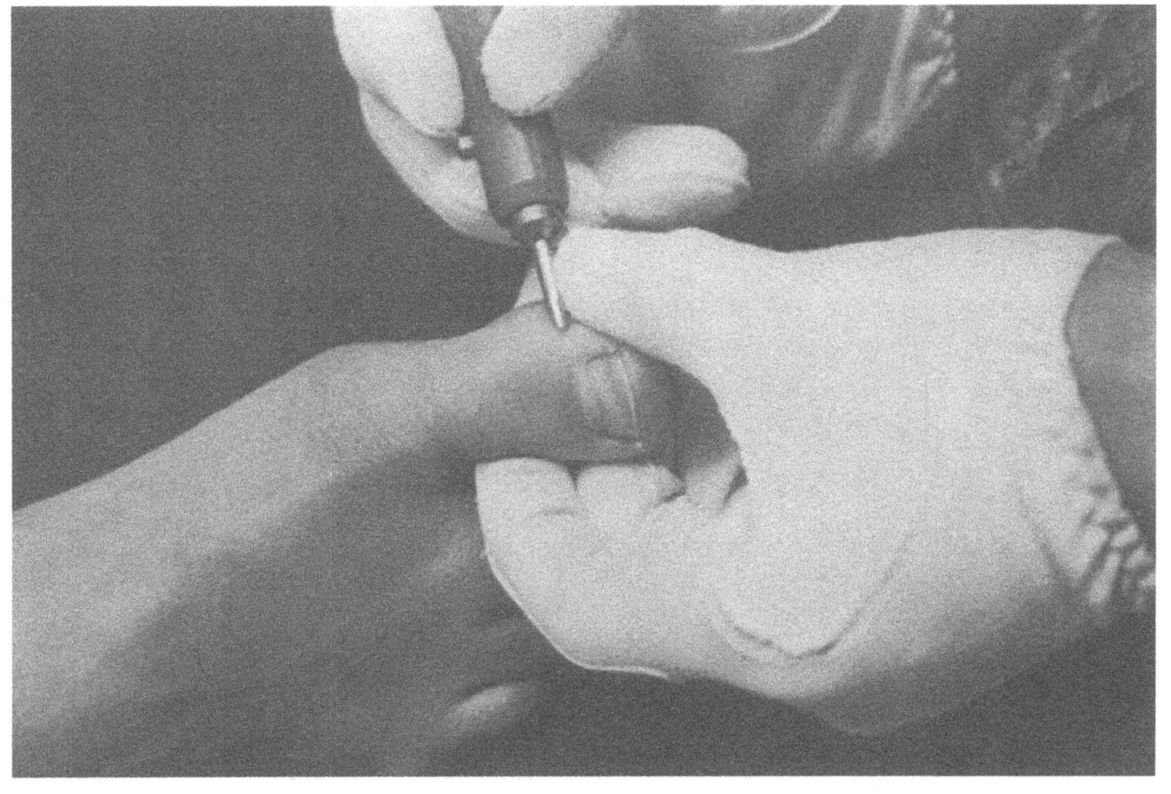

Pancreas — Right

4. MP-2 — Uric acid, high protein diet.

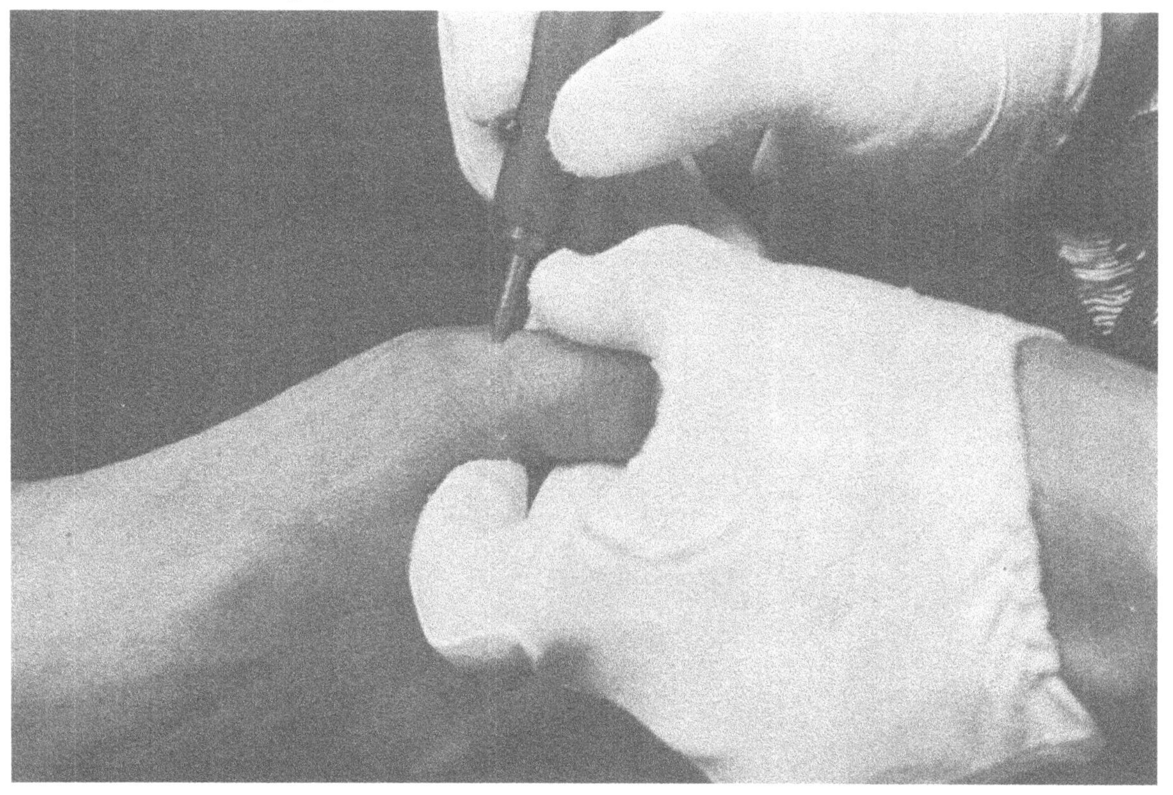

Pancreas — Right

5. MP-3 — CHO point.

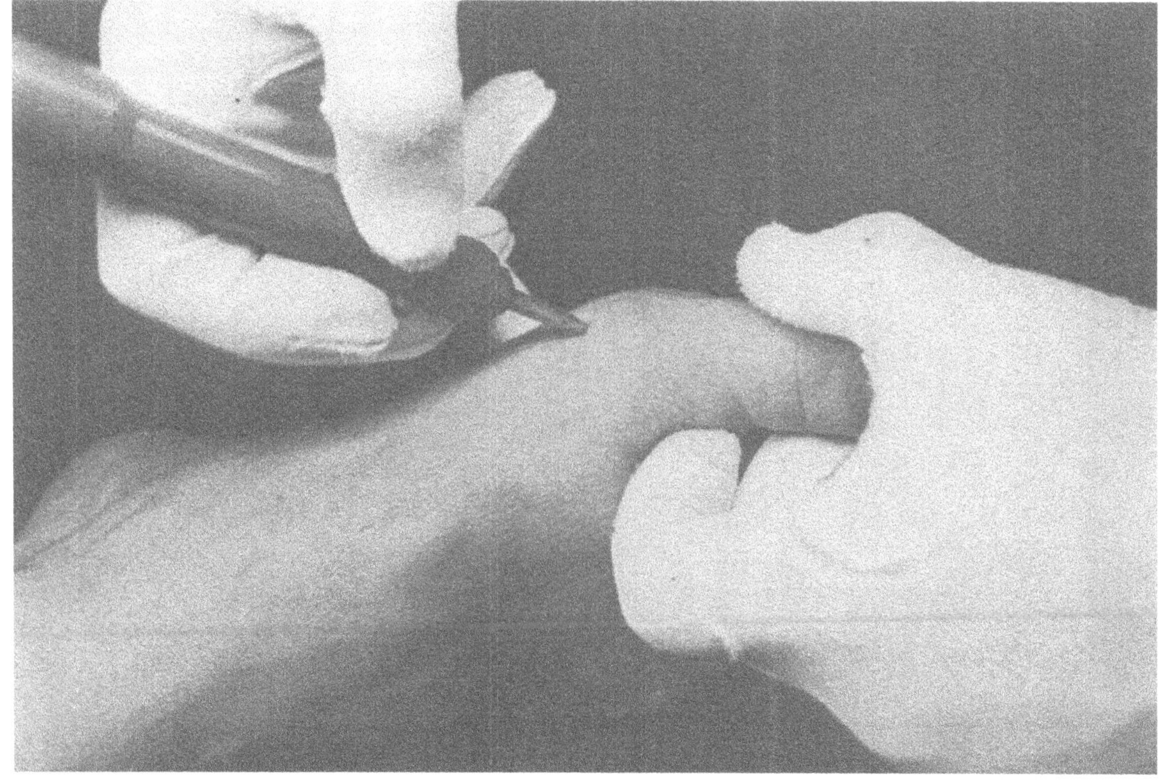

Pancreas — Right

6. MP-4 — Cholesterol, high lipase, fat metabolism.

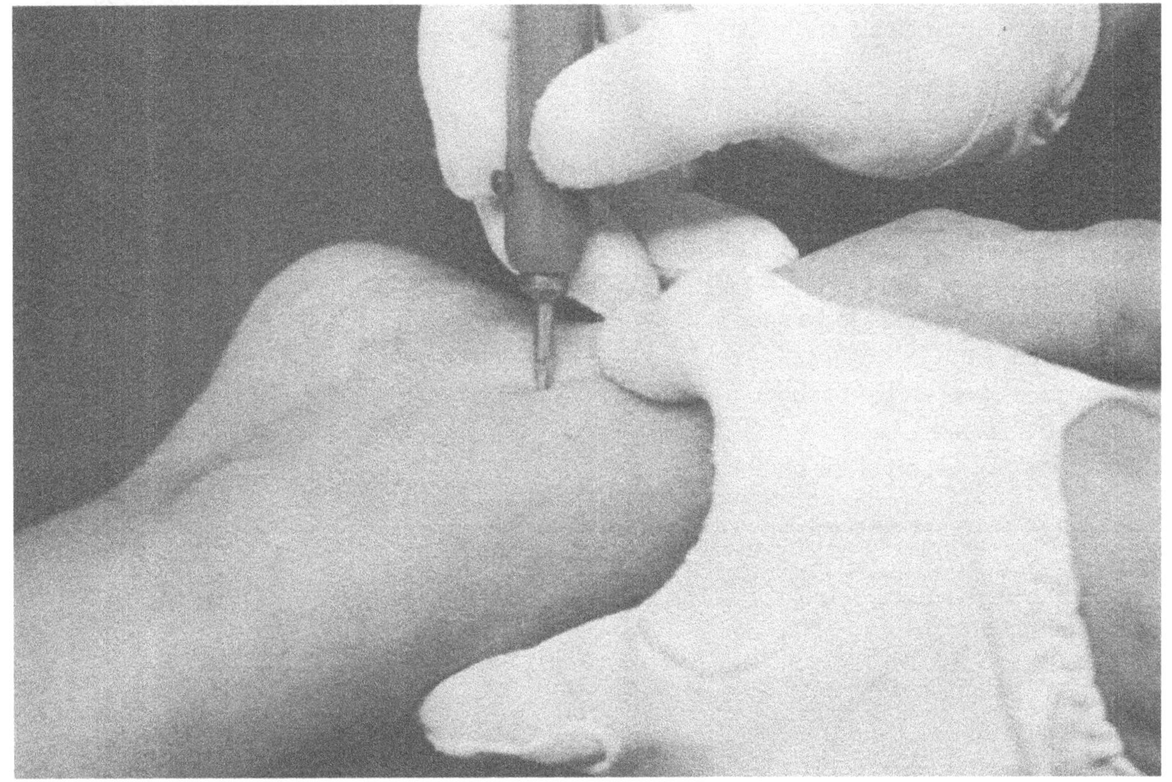

NOTES

Spleen — Left Side Only (drop here indicates allergy)

Voll's *Illustrated Volume II,* fig. 4, p. 17.

1. MP-1 — White pulp (foci of the upper portion of the body, neck and chest, insecticides, blood disease, white blood count).
2. CMP.
3. MP — Peritoneum.
4. MP-2 — White pulp (foci of the lower portion of body —abdomen and minor pelvis), memory point-mathematics with Li-MP-3, GV-MP-23-1-hippocampus.
5. MP-3 — Red pulp (pernicious anemia, polycythemia).
6. MP-4 — *Reticular endothelial system, immune system (defensive system). When finishing the Sp-CMP, always check Sp-MP-1 and 2; if you have all the foci under control and Sp-MP-4 immune system to balance it.*

Insecticides

1. Allergy 1 — Lower part of the body.
2. Liver 3 — Cirrhosis.
3. Spleen 2 — Lower part of the body.

NOTES

Spleen — Left

1. MP-1 — White pulp (foci of the upper portion of the body, neck and chest).

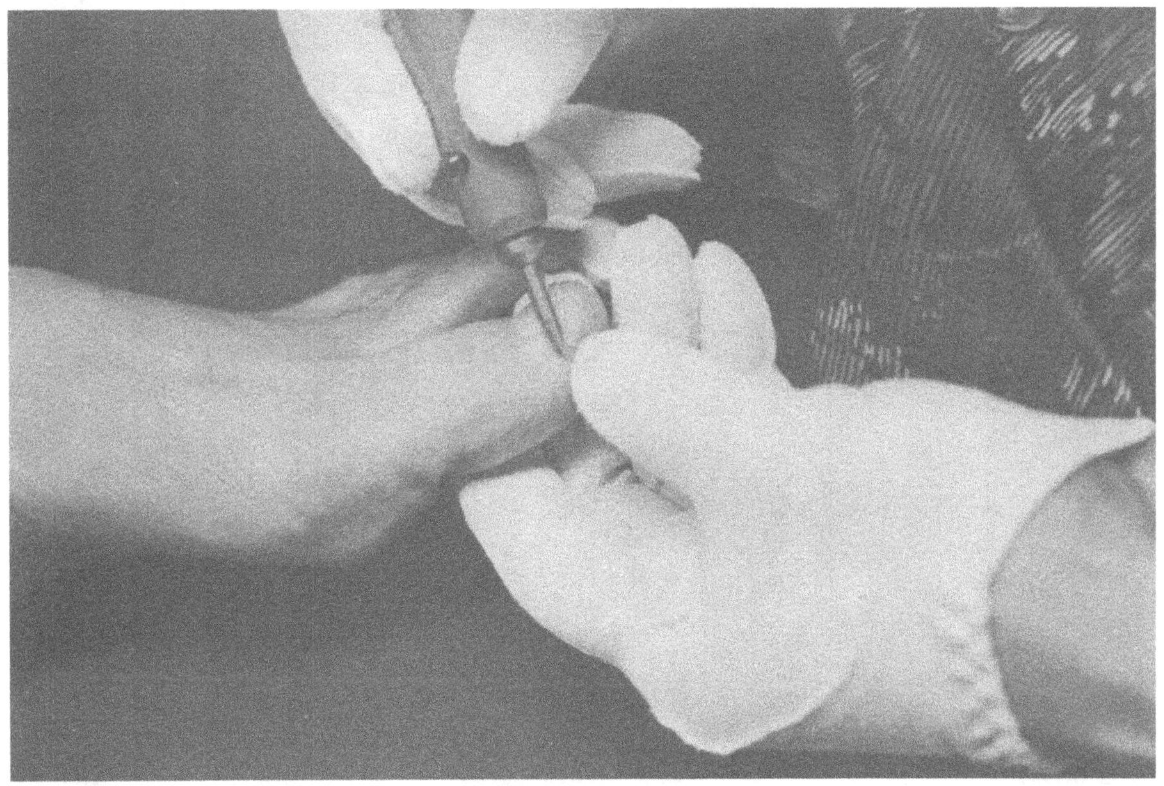

Spleen — Left

2. CMP.

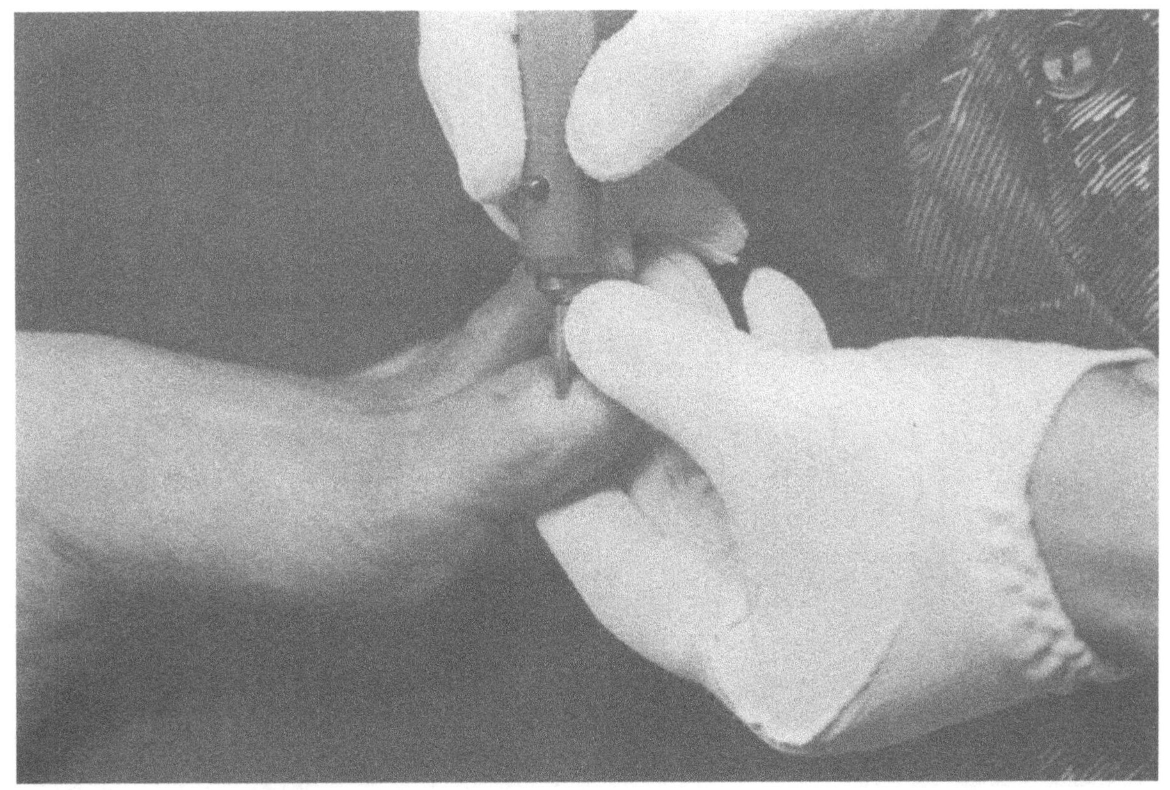

Spleen — Left

4. MP-2 — White pulp (foci of the lower portion of body — abdomen and minor pelvis).

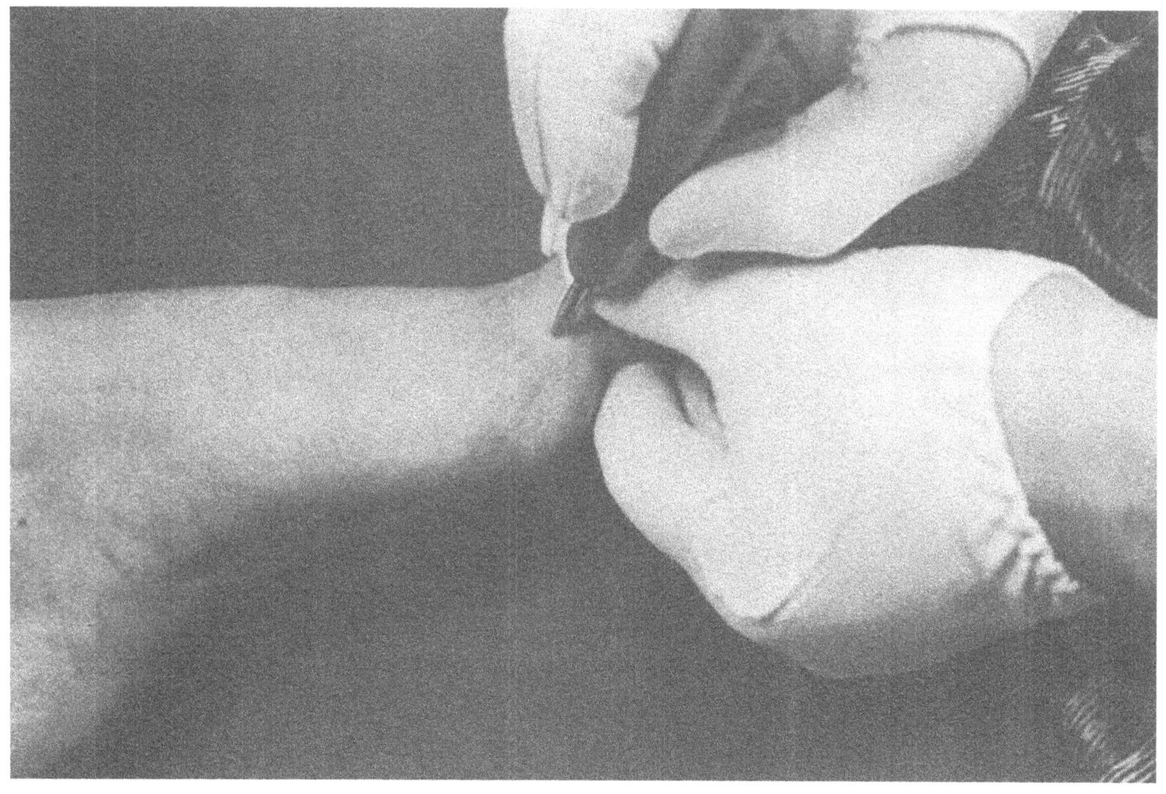

Spleen — Left

5. MP-3 — Red pulp (pernicious anemia, polycythemia).

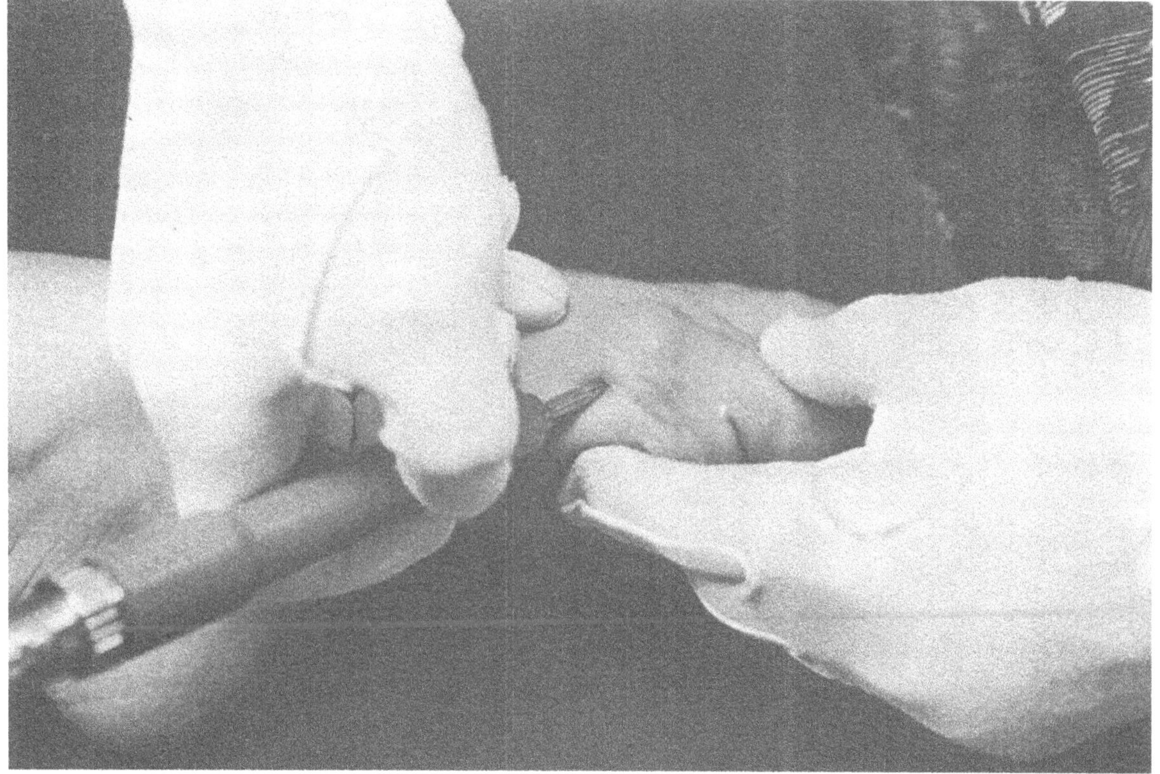

Spleen — Left

6. MP-4 — *Reticular endothelial system, immune system (defensive system).*

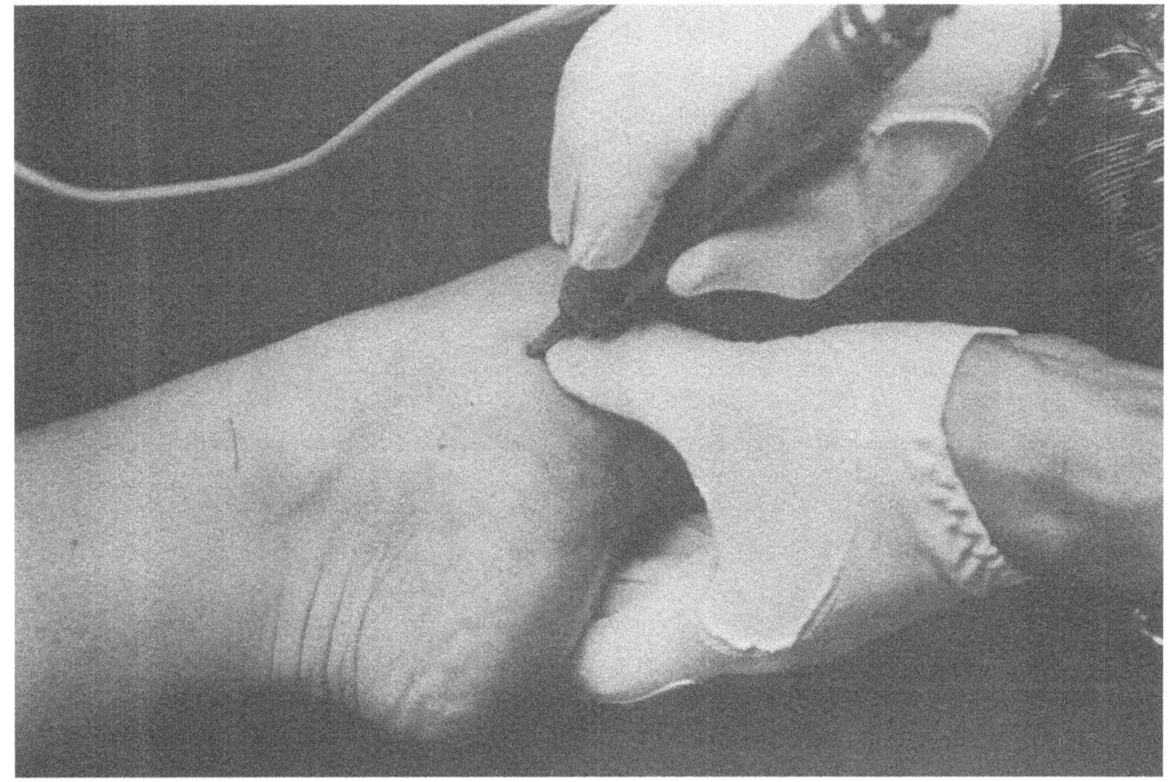

NOTES

Liver

Voll's *Illustrated Volume II,* fig. 12, p. 33.

May be influenced by lymphatic drainage of palatine tonsil Ly-1 and GV-20.

1. MP-1 — Portal vein, central venous system, stasis of portal veins.
2. CMP — Check vitamins (the acid citric cycle).
3. MP — Liver peritoneum.
4. MP-2 — Cirrhosis, bacteria, viruses (hepatitis), liver cell and lobular system.
5. MP-2a — Interlobular ducts.
6. MP-3 — Cirrhosis, perivascular system (chemical or pharmaceutical toxications, insecticides, alcohol intake, ID with Sp-MP-2), GV-23-1 for memory.
7. MP-7 — *Veins of lower extremities; check for thrombophlebitis (venous congestion), same side if vein ID on Ci-MP-8.*
8. MP-8 — *1st measurement point for knee joint*

NOTES

Liver

1. MP-1 — Portal vein, central venous system, stasis of portal veins.

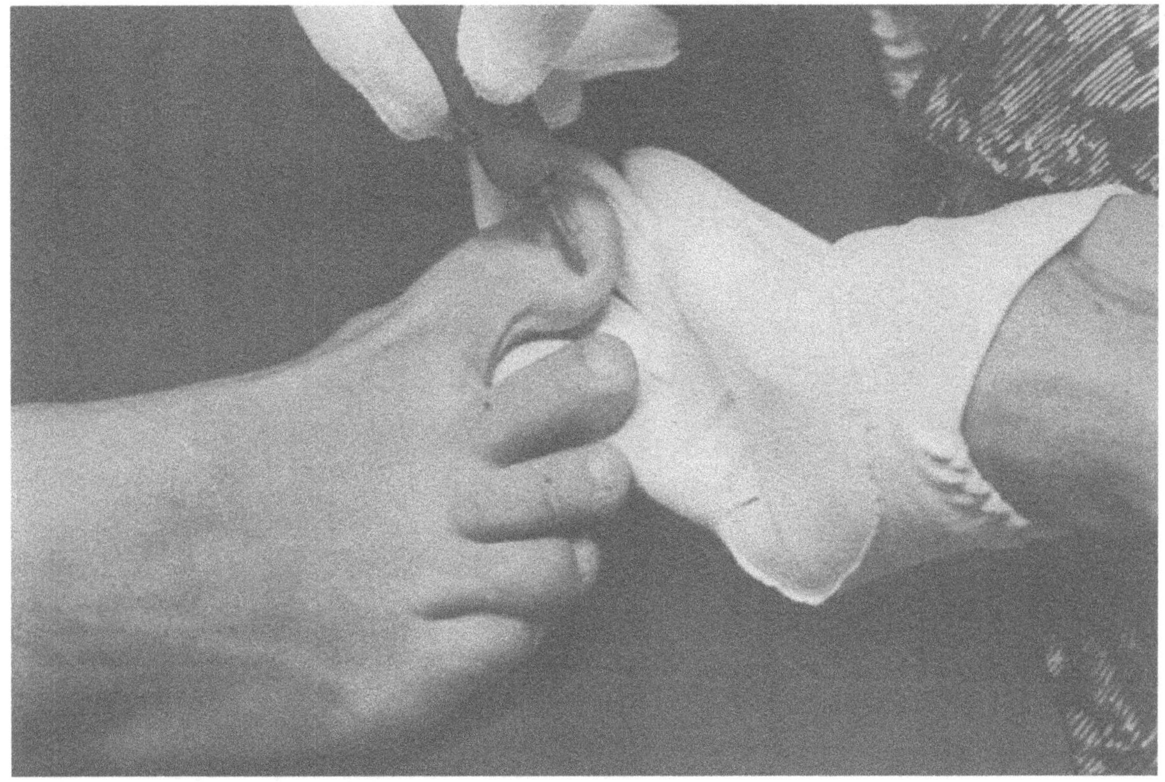

Liver

2. CMP — Check vitamins (the acid citric cycle).

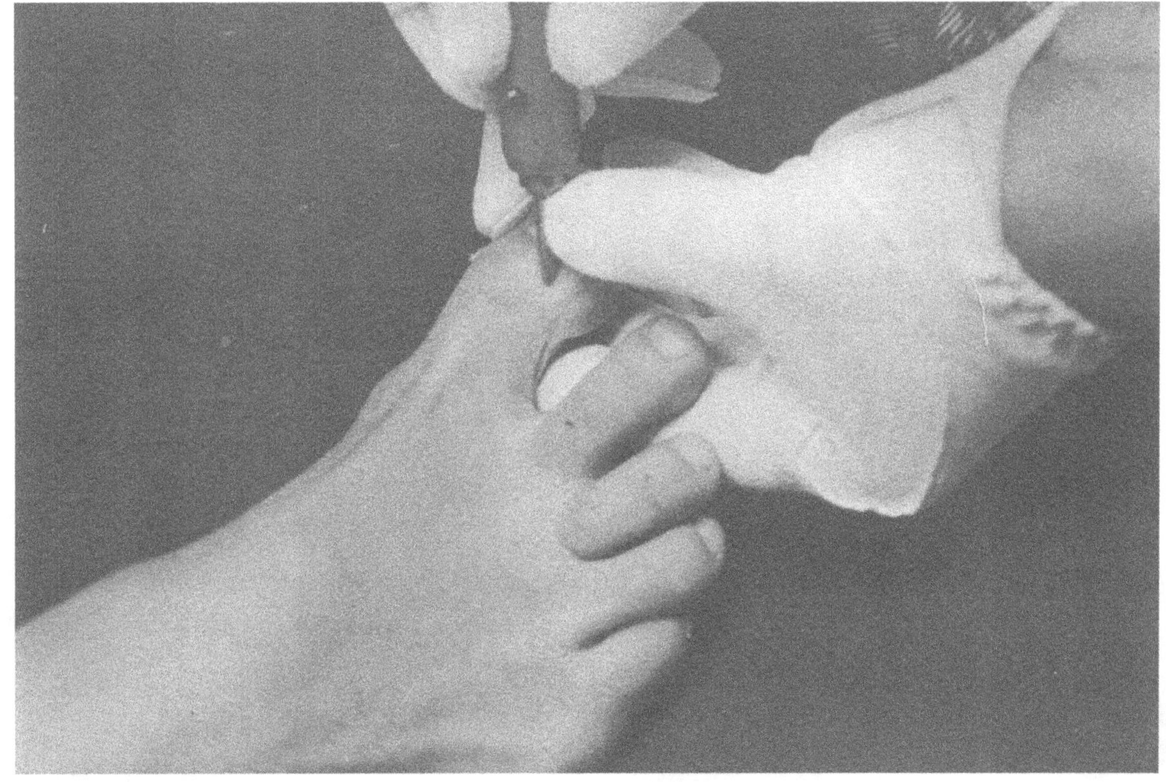

Liver

4. MP-2 — Cirrhosis, bacteria, viruses (hepatitis), liver cell and lobular system.

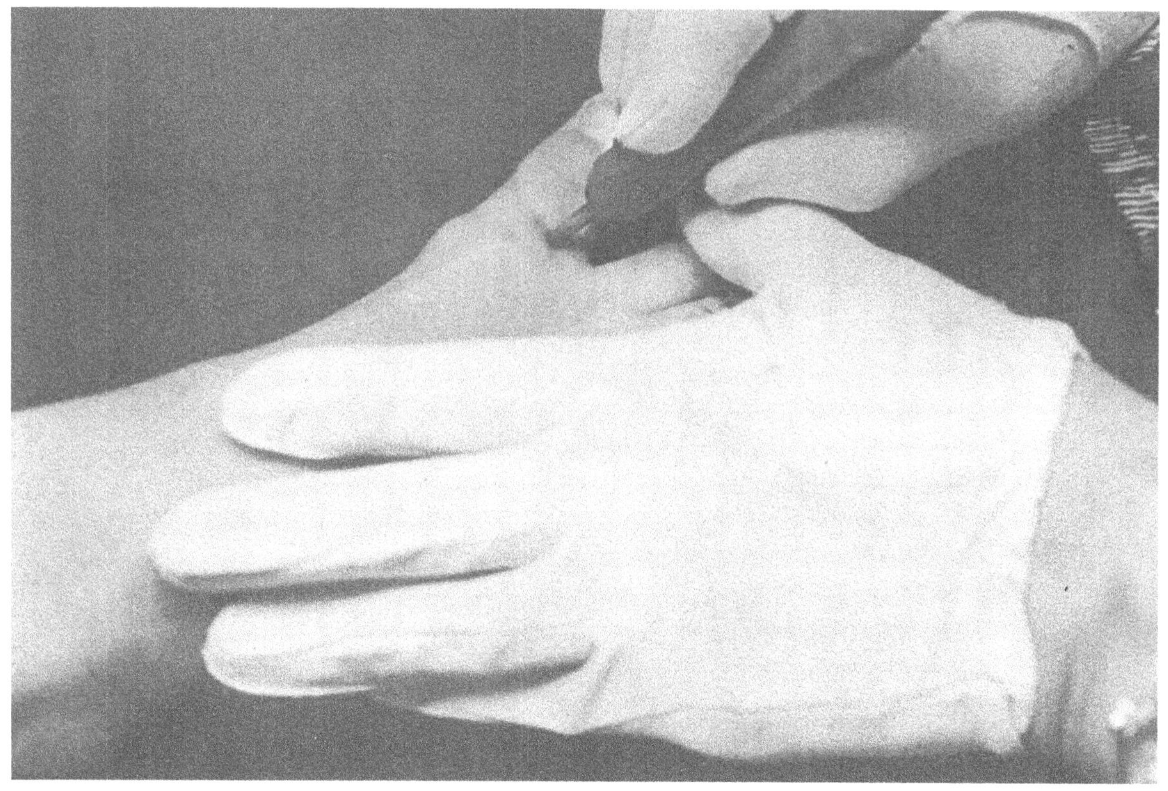

Liver

6. MP-3 — Cirrhosis, perivascular system.

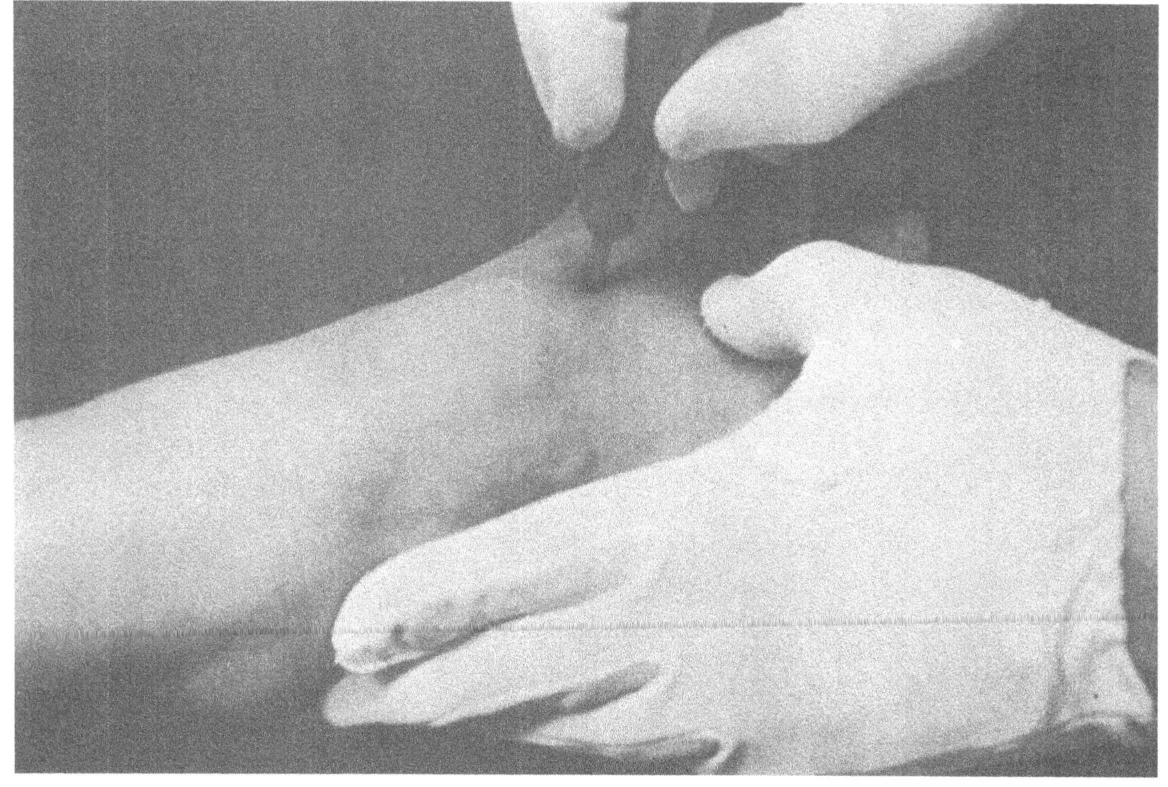

Joint Degeneration

Voll's *Illustrated Volume II,* fig. 32, p. 73.

1. MP-1 — All joints of the lower extremities, pelvic girdle.
2. CMP — All joints and spine.
3. MP — Synovial membranes for all joints (rheumatoid arthritis).
4. MP-2 — All joints of the upper extremities, shoulder girdle of the arm.
5. MP-3 — TMJ, 1st and 2nd cervicals.

NOTES

Joint Degeneration

1. MP-1 — All joints of the lower extremities, pelvic girdle.

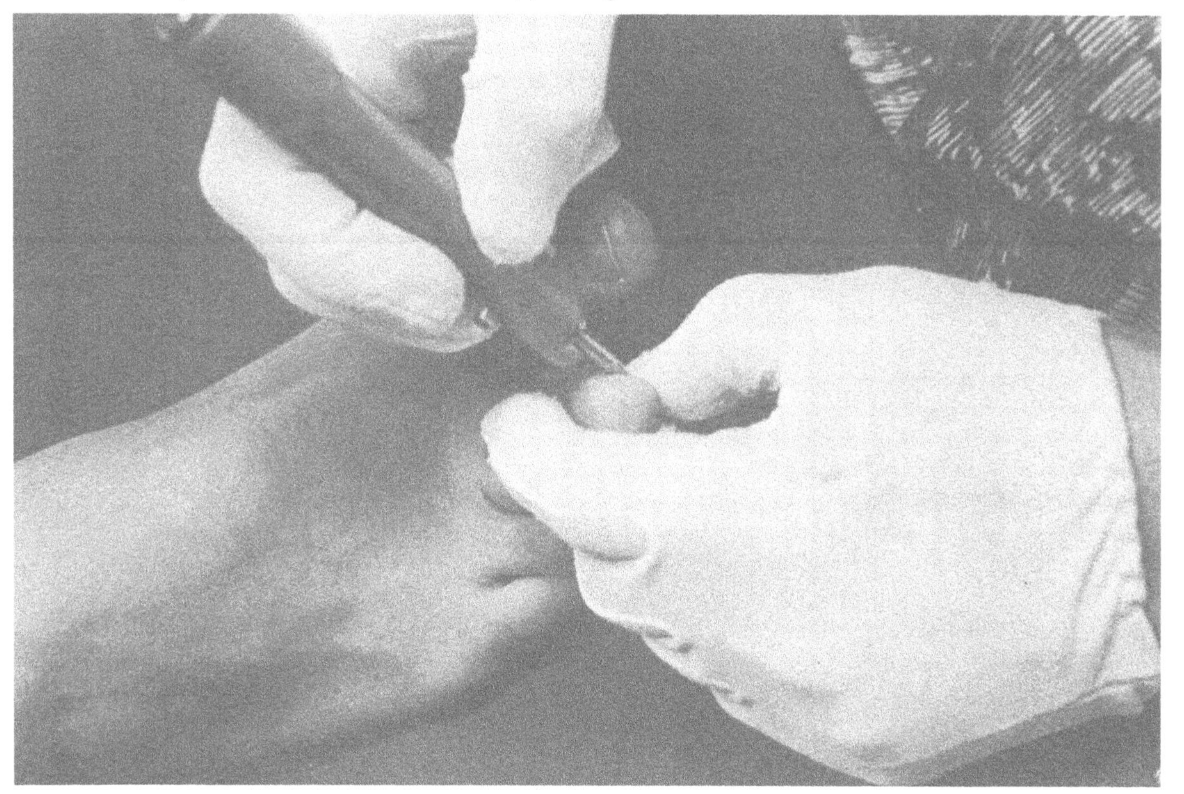

Joint Degeneration

2. CMP — All joints and spine.

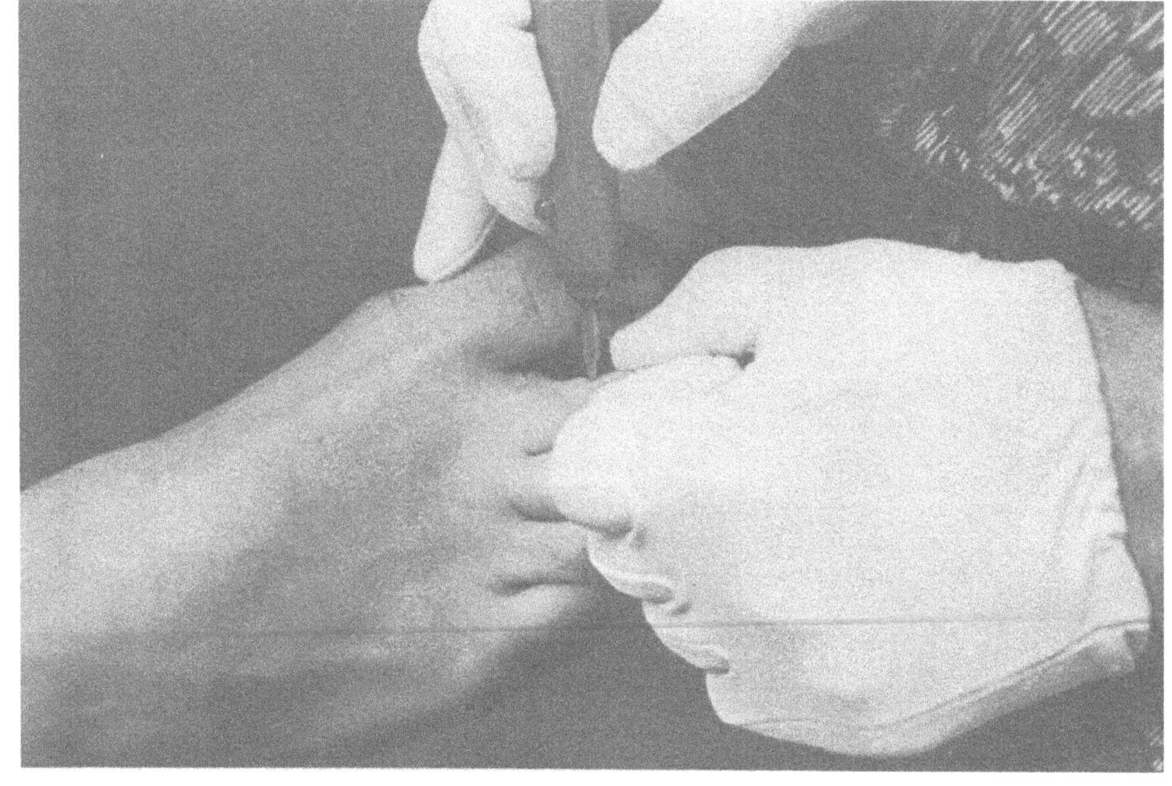

Joint Degeneration

3. MP — Synovial membranes for all joints (rheumatoid arthritis).

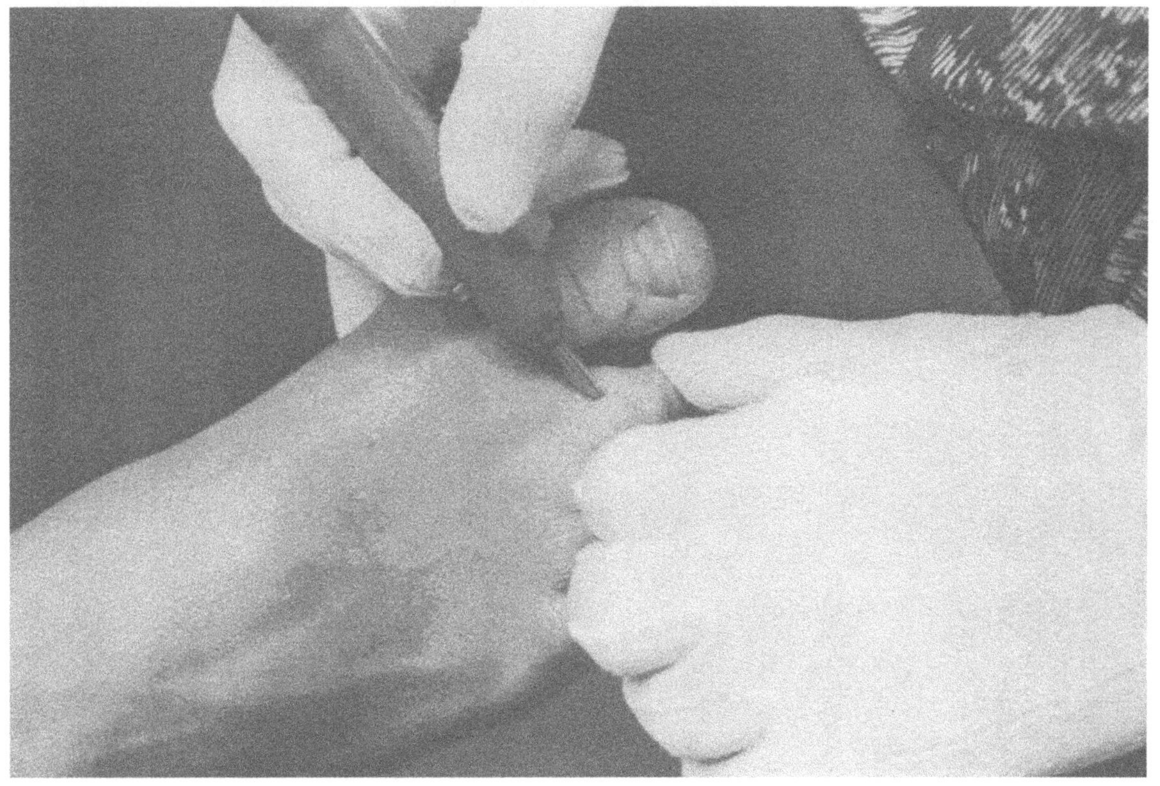

Joint Degeneration

4. MP-2 — All joints of the upper extremities, shoulder girdle of the arm.

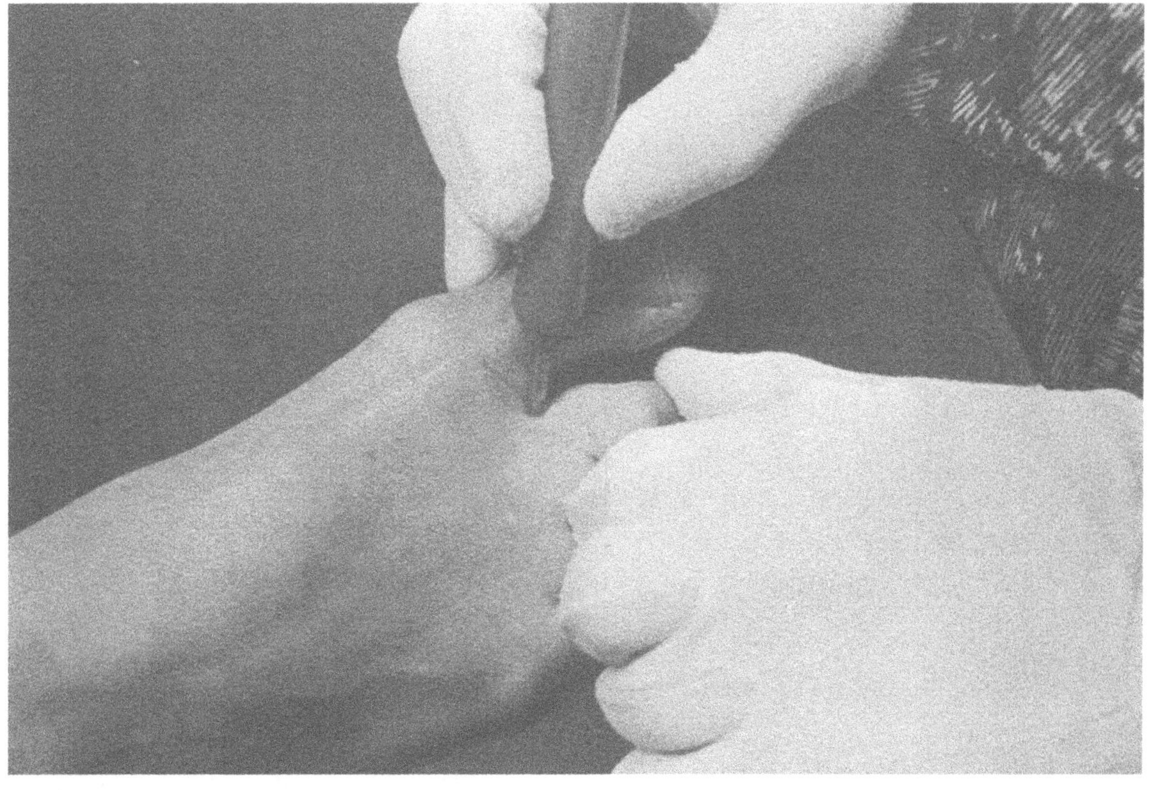

Joint Degeneration

5. MP-3 — TMJ, 1st and 2nd cervicals.

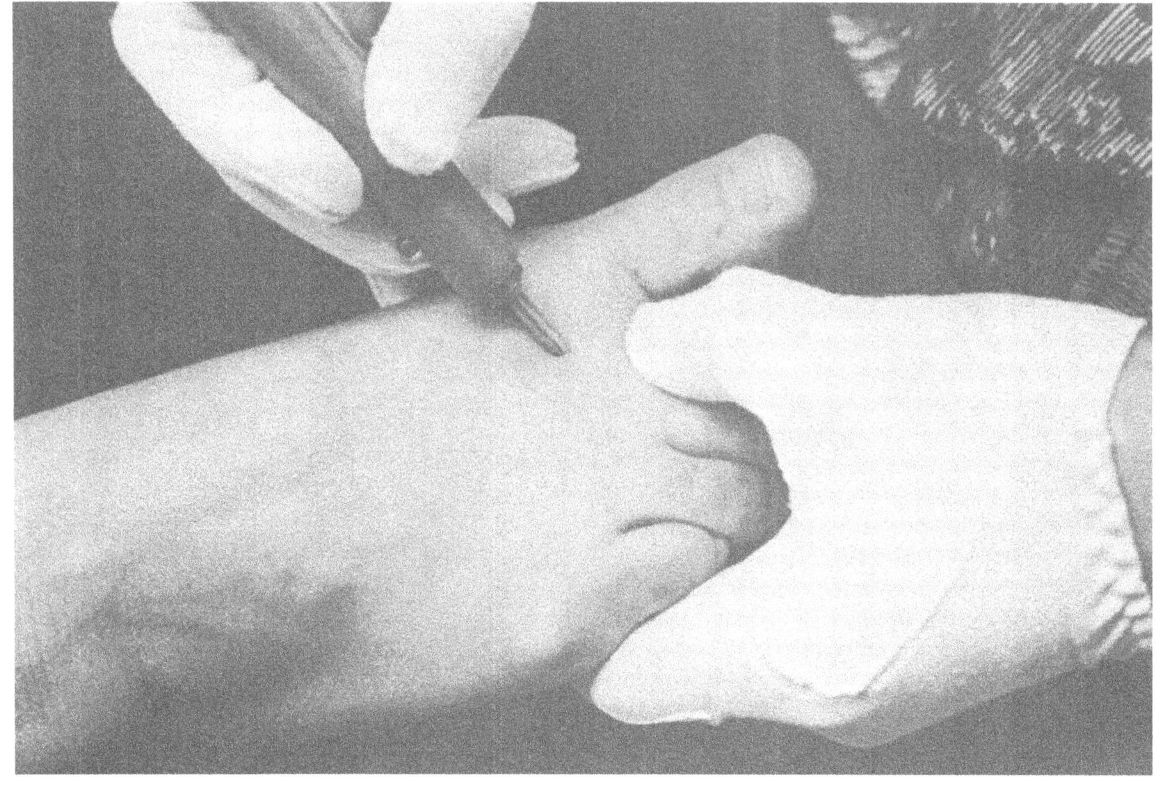

NOTES

Stomach

Voll's *Illustrated Volume II,* fig. 8a, p. 24; fig. 8b, p. 25.

1. MP-45 — Left MP of body of stomach, right MP of pyloric.
2. Celiac plexus 44-C HCL, mint (right side), coffee (left side).
   Textual and Illustrated Volume III, figs. 12,13, pp. 126,127.
   Celiac plexus 44-C Stomach — if ID:
   a. *MP-SI-1a — Upper mesenteric plexus.*
   b. *MP-St-19 — Phrenic plexus.*
   c. *MP-St-22 — Upper gastric plexus (on right side only).*
   d. *MP-Ki-21 — Hepatic branches of the vagus nerve.*
   e. *MP-GBL-43-C — Hepatic plexus.*
   f. *MP-Ki-1-1 — Renal plexus.*
   g. *MP-Ki-1b — Suprarenal plexus.*
3. CMP —Stomach.
4. *St-44a — Stomach peritoneum.*
5. *MP-43a — St. tract right ascending part; St. tract left descending tract.*
6. *MP-43 — Cardia (left) Pyloric (right); body of St. for the short part ascending to pars.*
7. *MP-Esophagus — St-42a lower portion (midline pain).*
8. *MP-Esophagus — St-42 upper portion.*
9. *MP-41a — Mammary gland it ID on MP-TW mammary gland. Affects endocrine gland: (St-MP-9 parathyroid, St-MP-10 thyroid, St-MP-11 thymus) — check for spine, ligament and infection problems. St-MP-31 gonad, St-MP-2 TMJ, lower part (jaw ostitis).*
10. *MP-33 — Abdominal veins (if ID on circulation MP-8, thrombophlebitis).*
11. *MP-32 — Arteries of leg (smoker's leg — upper leg, anterior view if ID on circulation MP-9).*
12. *MP-31, Sp-Pa-11, LI-11 — Gonads.*
13. MP-Stomach 12 — Carotid sinus, common carotid artery.
    Textual and Illustrated Volume III, figs. 24, 25, pp. 144, 145.
    a. *MP-GBL-20 — Sympathetic nerve.*
    b. *MP-TW-1a — Cervical ganglia of sympathetic nerve.*
    c. *MP-Circulation 8e — Thoracic aortic plexus.*
    d. *MP-Circulation 9 — Arteries.*
    e. *MP-Ki-1b — Suprarenal plexus.*
    f. *MP-Ki-1-1 — Renal plexus.*
14. *MP-4 — Sphenoid sinus (may affect high blood pressure because it is related to the cavernous sinus. Cavernous sinus has internal carotid arteries with sympathetics).*

NOTES

Stomach

1. MP-45 — Left MP of body of stomach, right MP of pyloric.

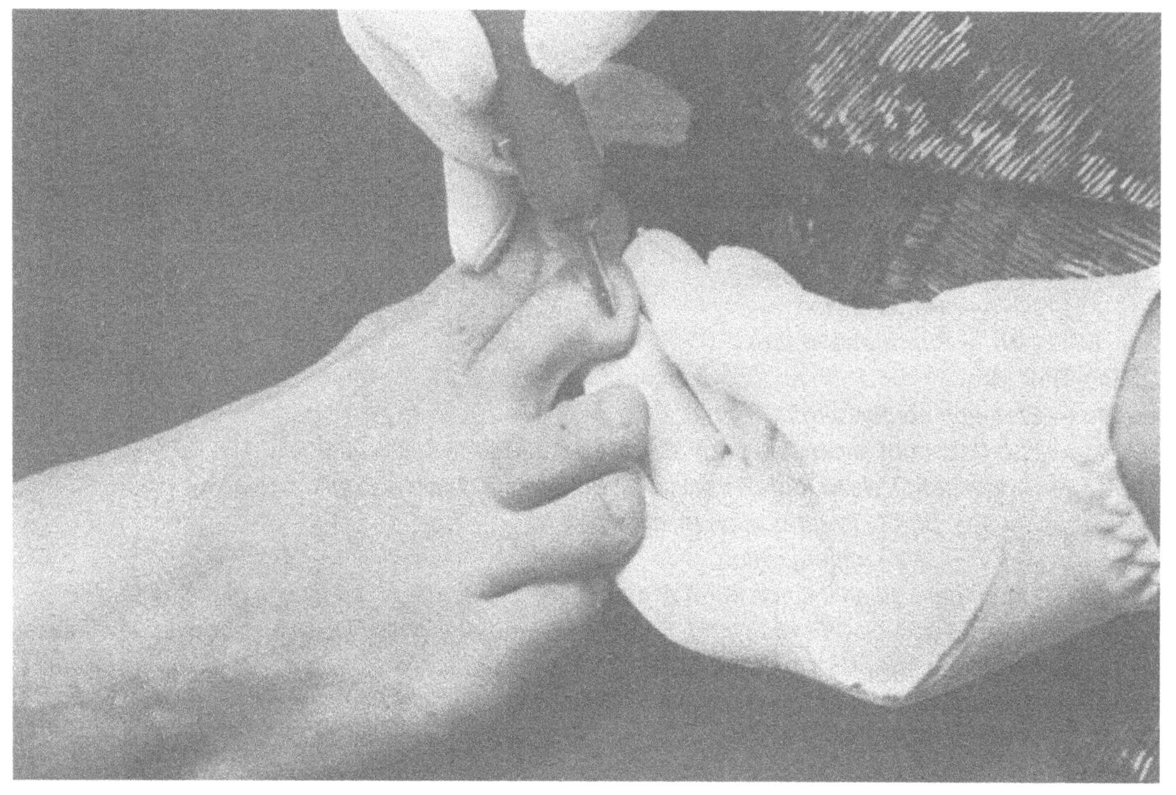

Stomach

2. Celiac plexus 44-C — HCL, mint (right side), coffee (left side).

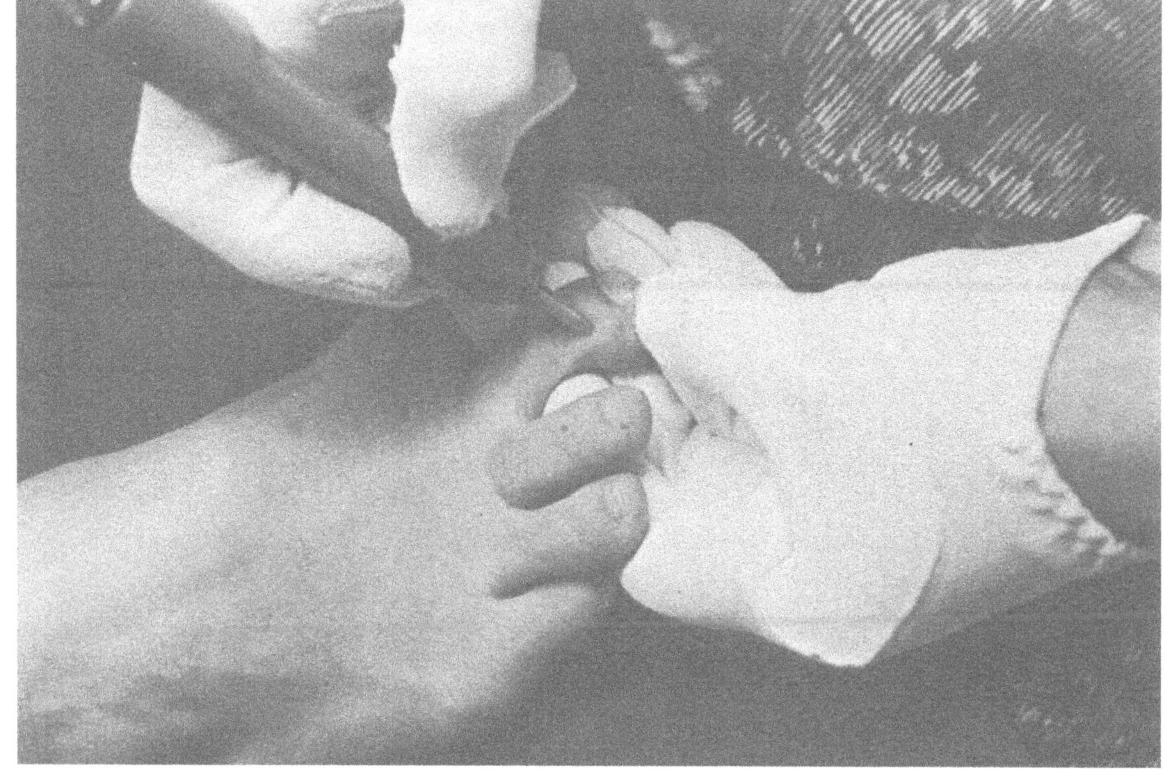

Stomach

3. CMP — Stomach.

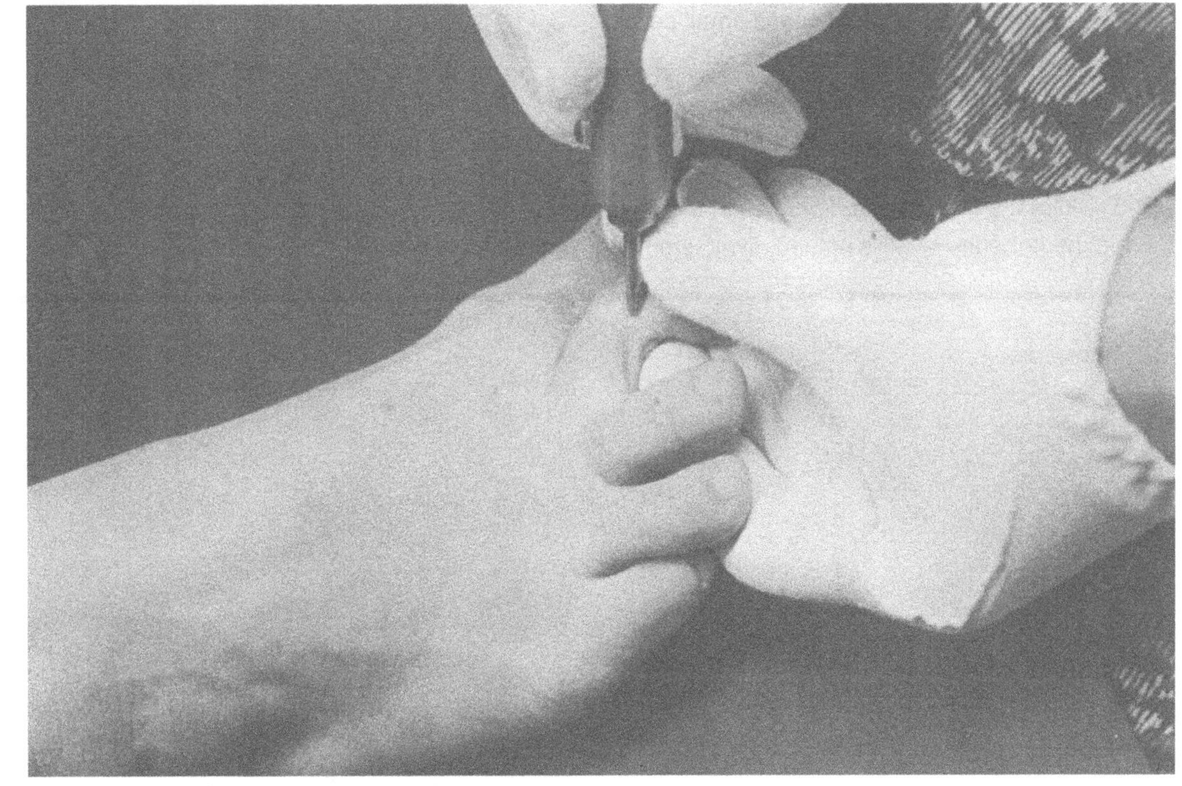

NOTES

Fibroid Degeneration (Tri-part div.)

Voll's *Illustrated Volume II,* fig. 29, p. 65.

Fibroid degeneration attacks do not permit the cell to carry out its normal function.

1. MP-1 — Organs of the abdomen and small pelvis.
2. CMP — 1st fibroid degeneration of whole body.
3. CMP — 2nd mucous membrane.
4. MP-2 — Organs of chest and neck, breast, heart (check with St-41a for fibrocystic disease and fibromatosis of mammary gland).
5. MP-3 — Organs of the head, fibromas in the nasal sinus.
6. Fibroid peritoneum — MPs spleen, liver, stomach, gallbladder, bladder, kidney.

NOTES

Fibroid Degeneration

1. MP-1 — Organs of the abdomen and small pelvis.

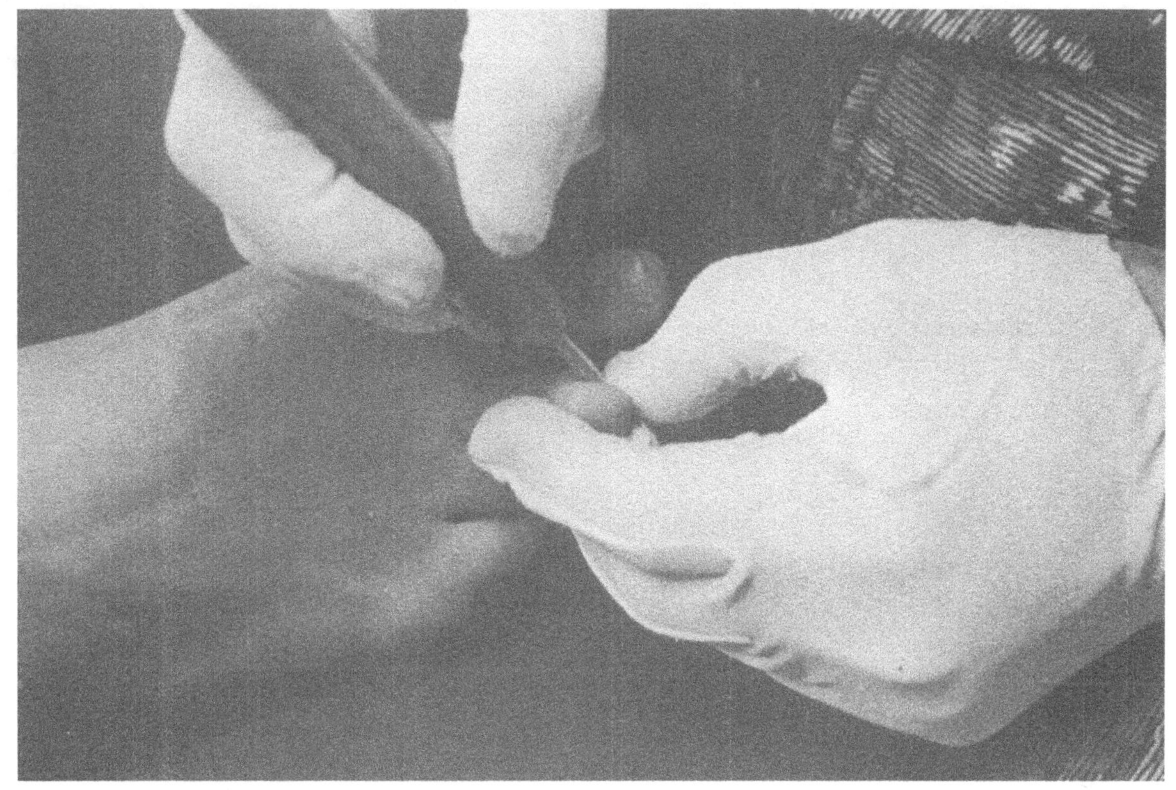

Fibroid Degeneration

2. CMP — 1st fibroid degeneration of whole body.

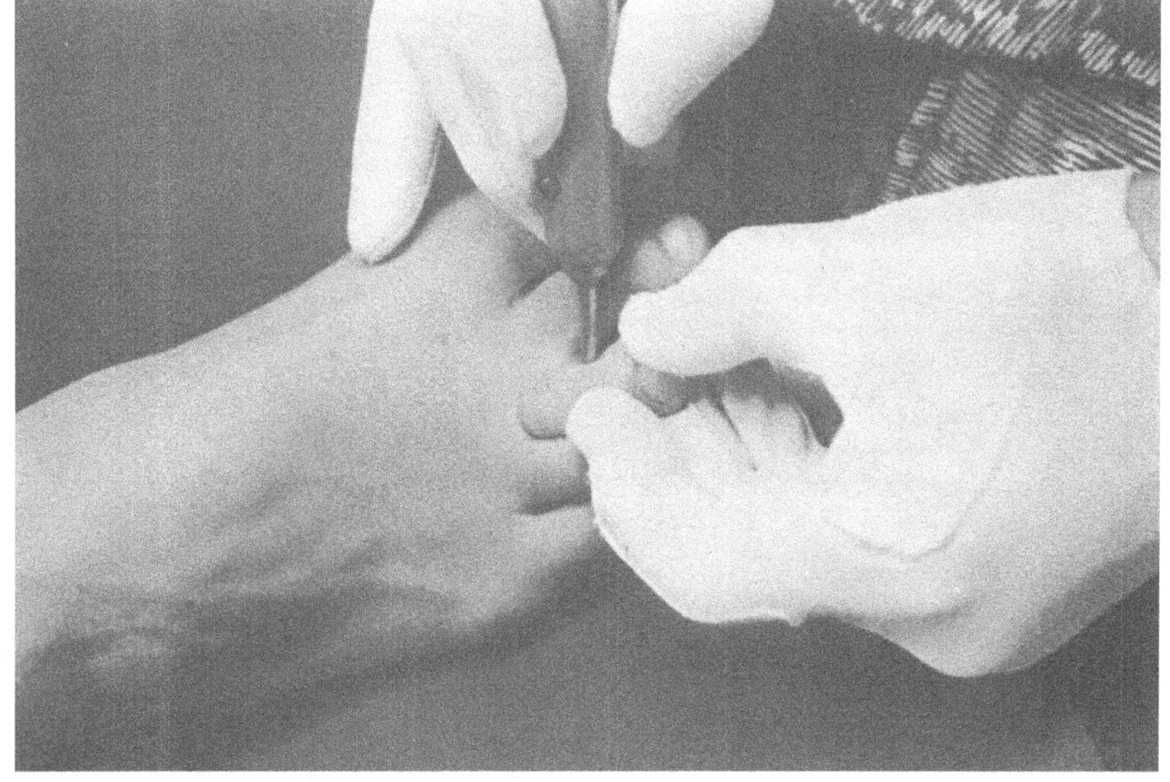

Fibroid Degeneration

4. MP-2 — Organs of chest and neck, breast, heart.

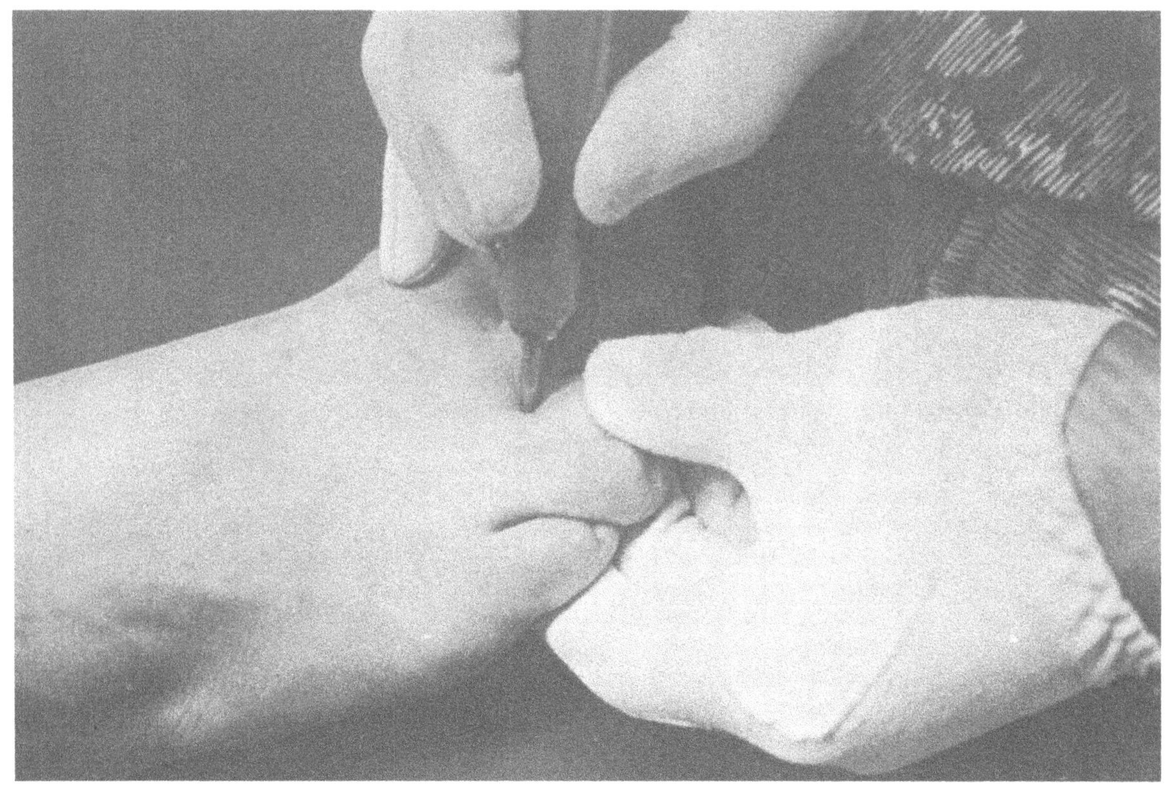

Fibroid Degeneration

5. MP-3 — Organs of the head, fibromas in the nasal sinus.

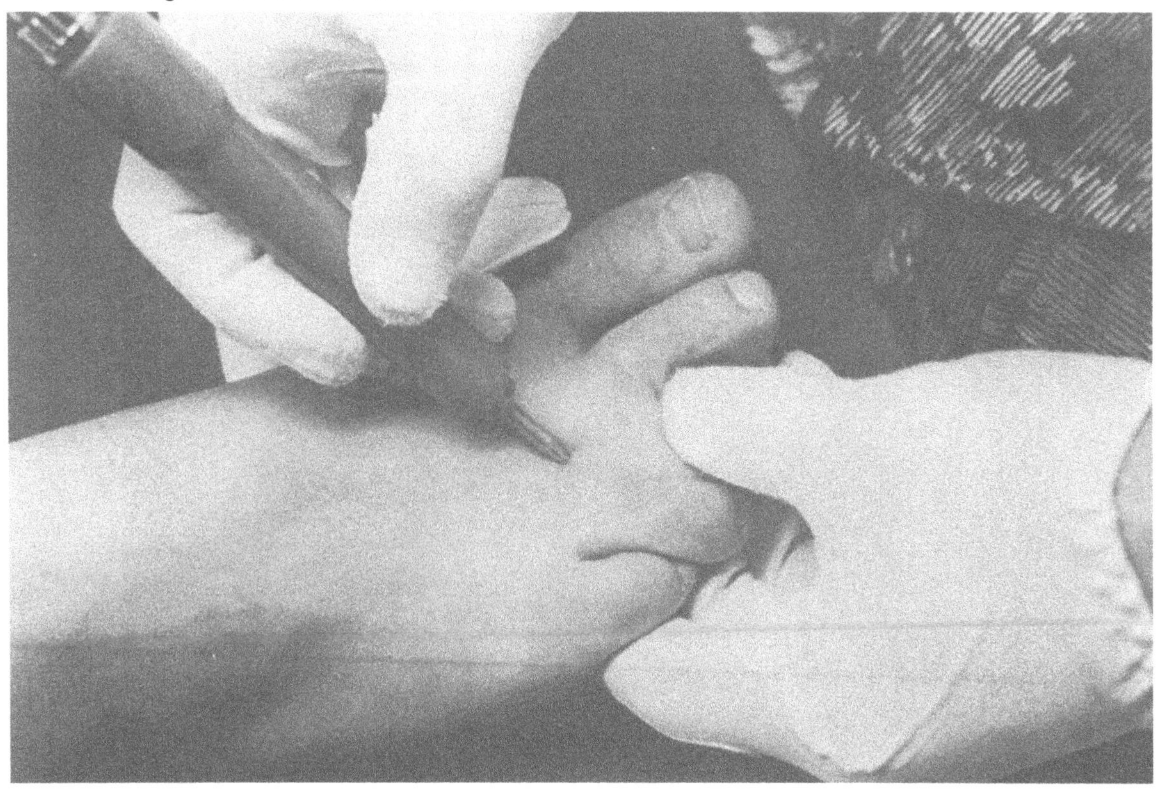

Skin (Tri-part div.)

Voll's *Illustrated Volume II*, fig. 20, p. 49.
Diagnosis for allergies.

1. MP-1 — Skin of the lower portion of body.
2. MP — Scars, skin of the whole body.
3. MP-2 — Skin, upper portion of the body.
4. MP-3 — Skin of the head.

NOTES

Skin

1. MP-1 — Skin of the lower portion of body.

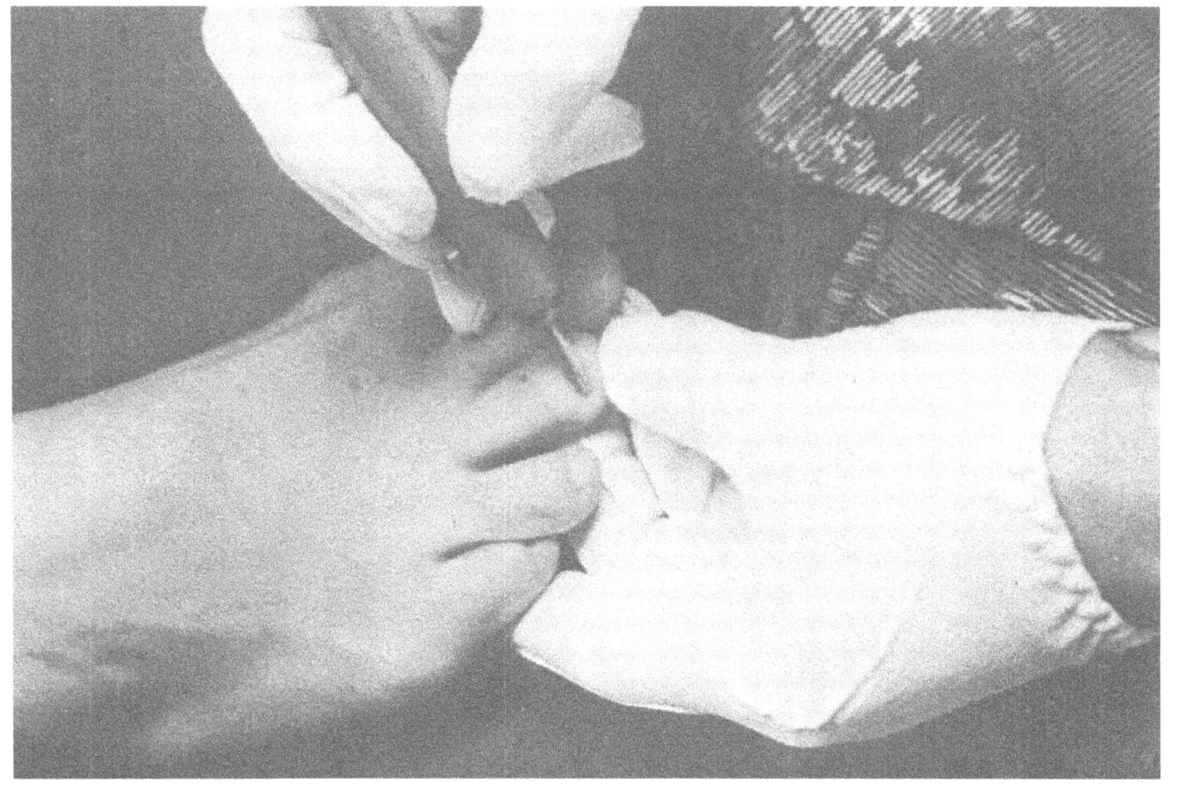

Skin

2. MP — Scars, skin of the whole body.

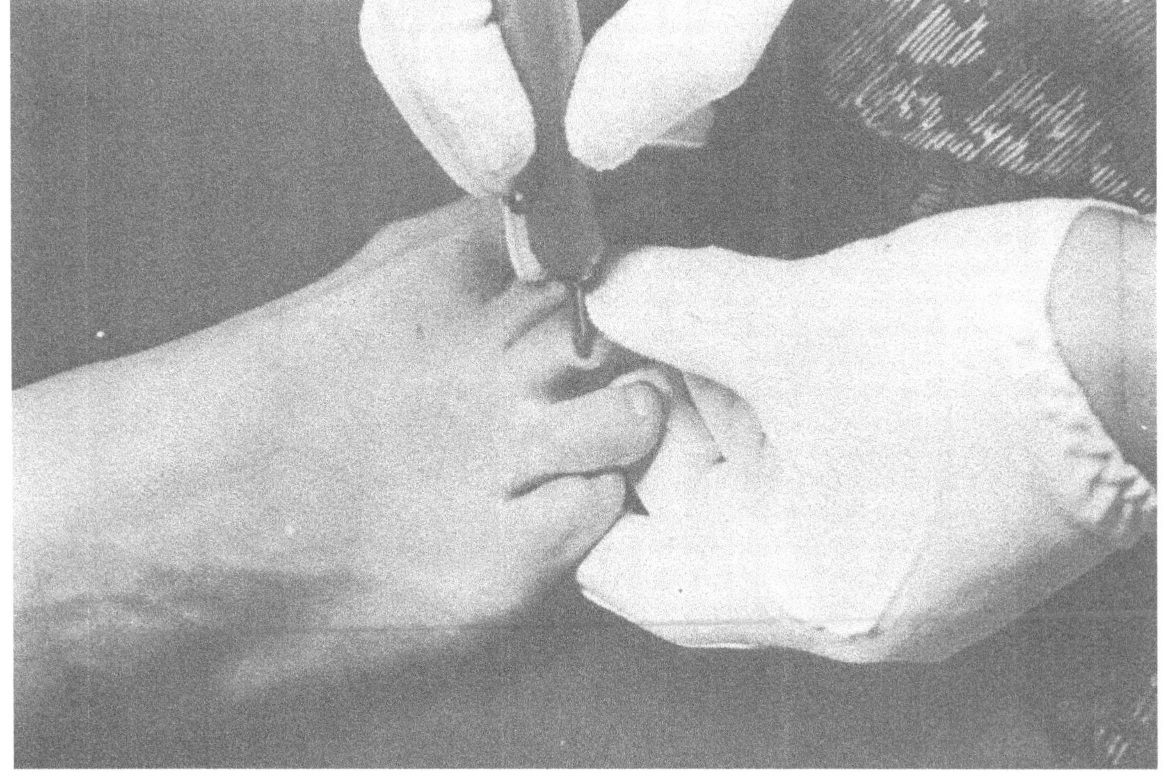

Skin

3. MP-2 — Skin, upper portion of the body.

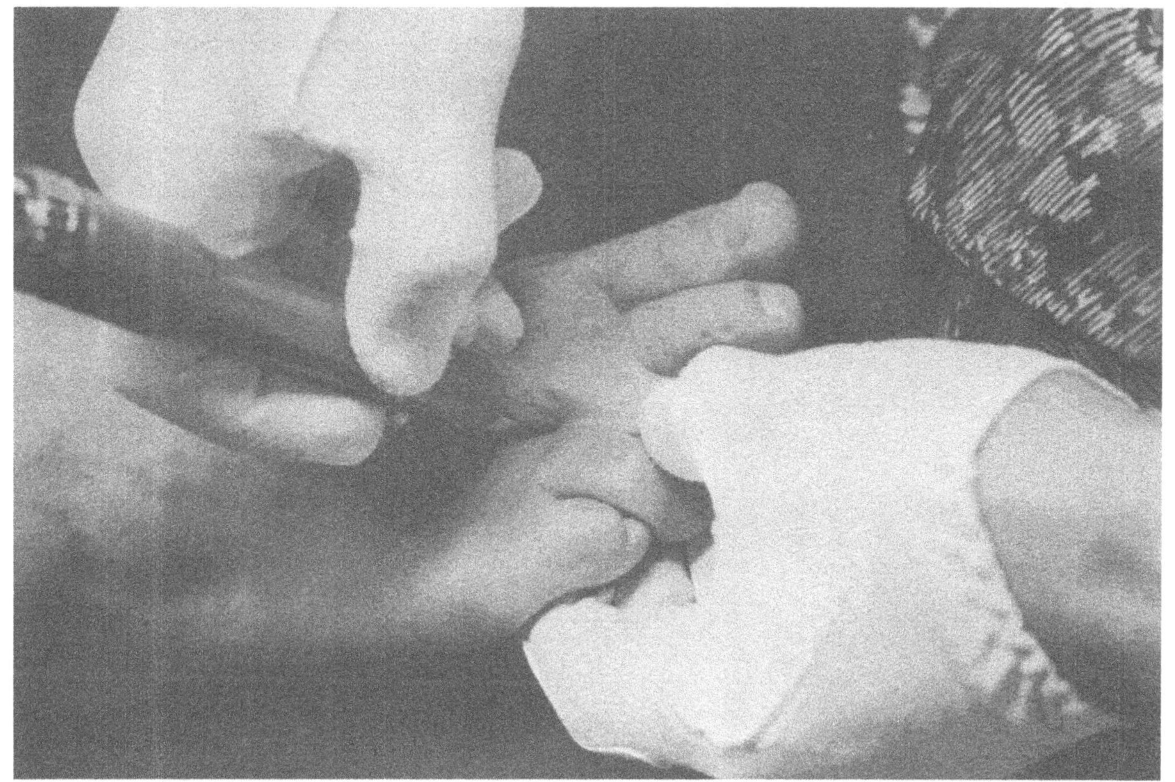

Skin

4. MP-3 — Skin of the head.

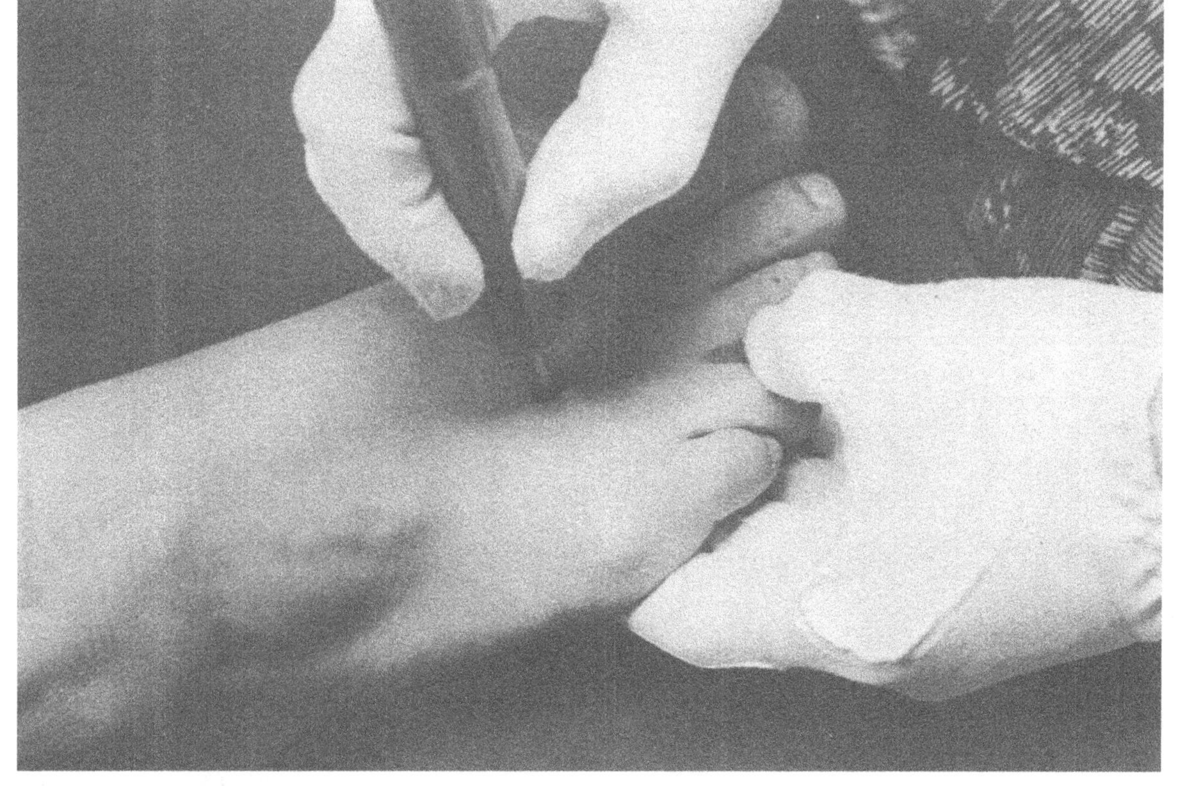

Fatty Degeneration

Voll's *Illustrated Volume II,* fig. 29, p. 67.
If ID, check Pa-4.

1. MP-1 — Fatty degeneration of organs in the abdomen, lower body — liver, kidney, lipoidnephrosis, lipomatosis of the pancreas.
2. CMP — Fatty degeneration of whole body (compare with Pa-MP-4).
3. MP-2 — Of organs and vessels in the chest (fatty heart muscles, coronary vessels, arteries).
4. MP-3 — Organs and vessels in the head, brain, cerebral malacia, cerebral sclerosis (check allergy MP-3, also organ degeneration MP-3).

NOTES

Fatty Degeneration

1. MP-1 — Fatty degeneration of organs in the abdomen, lower body.

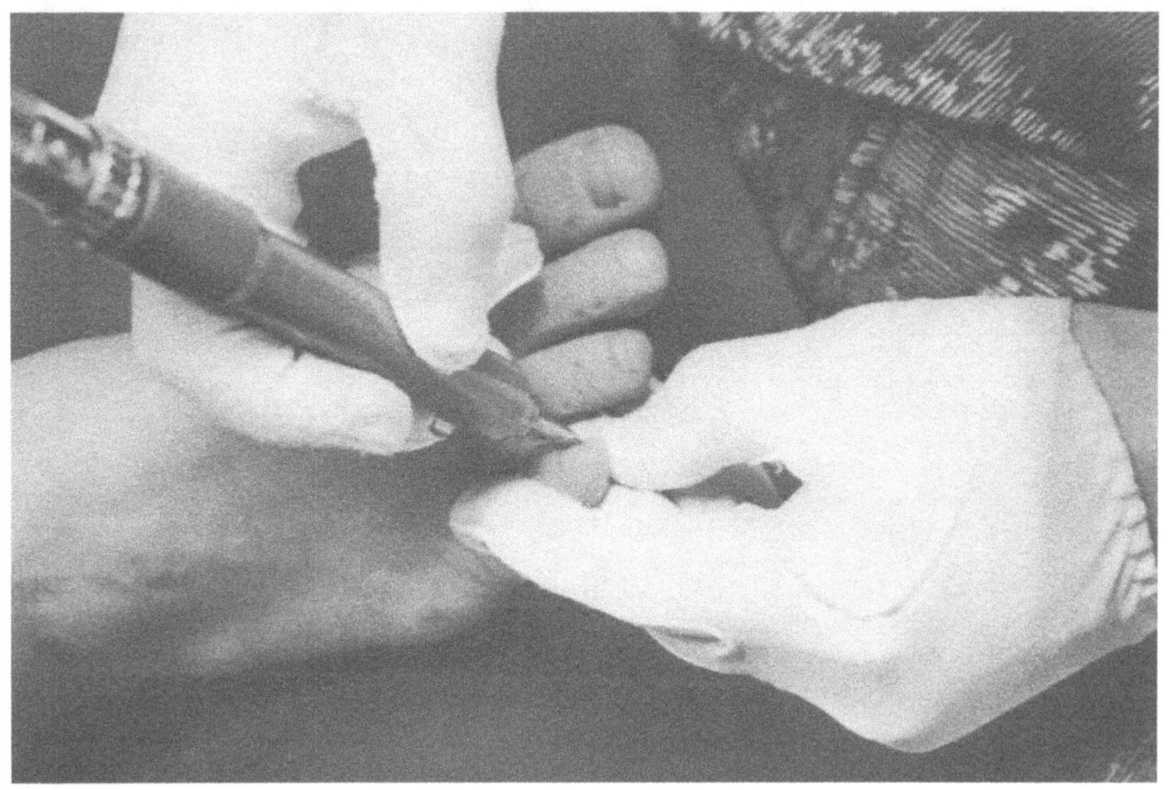

Fatty Degeneration

2. CMP — Fatty degeneration of whole body.

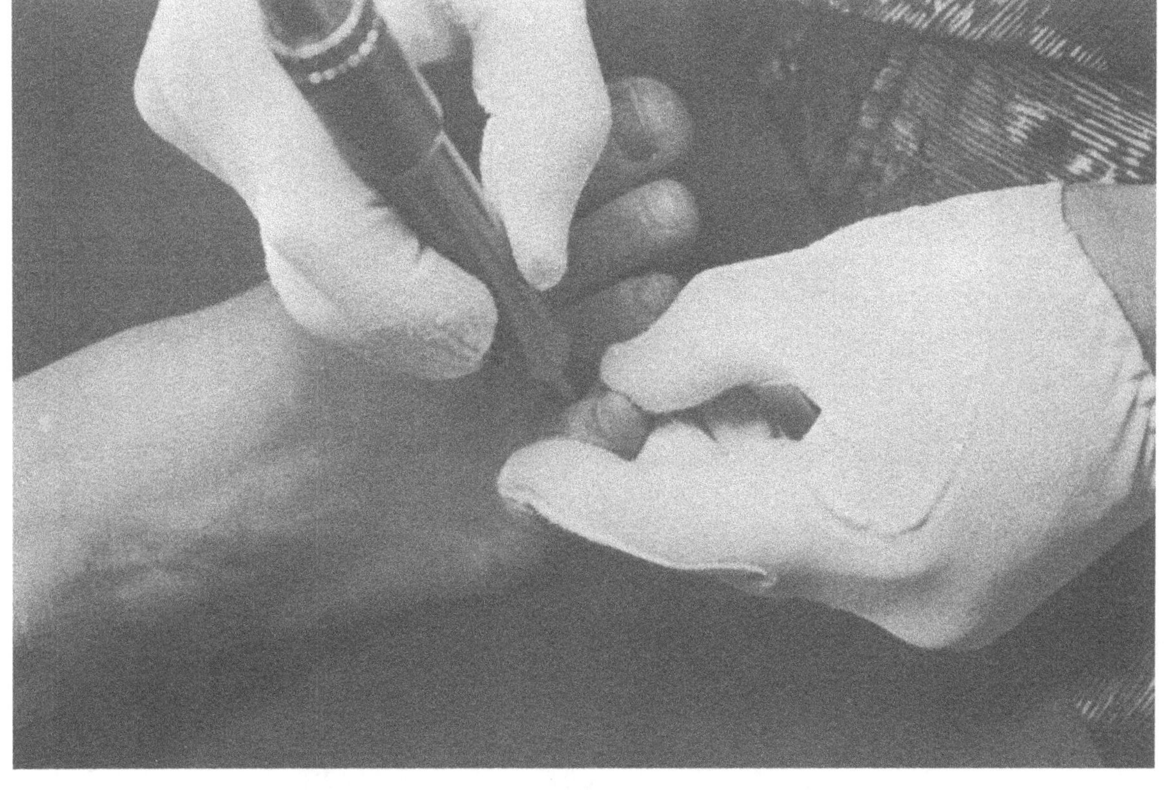

Fatty Degeneration

3. MP-2 — Of organs and vessels in the chest (fatty heart muscles, coronary vessels, arteries).

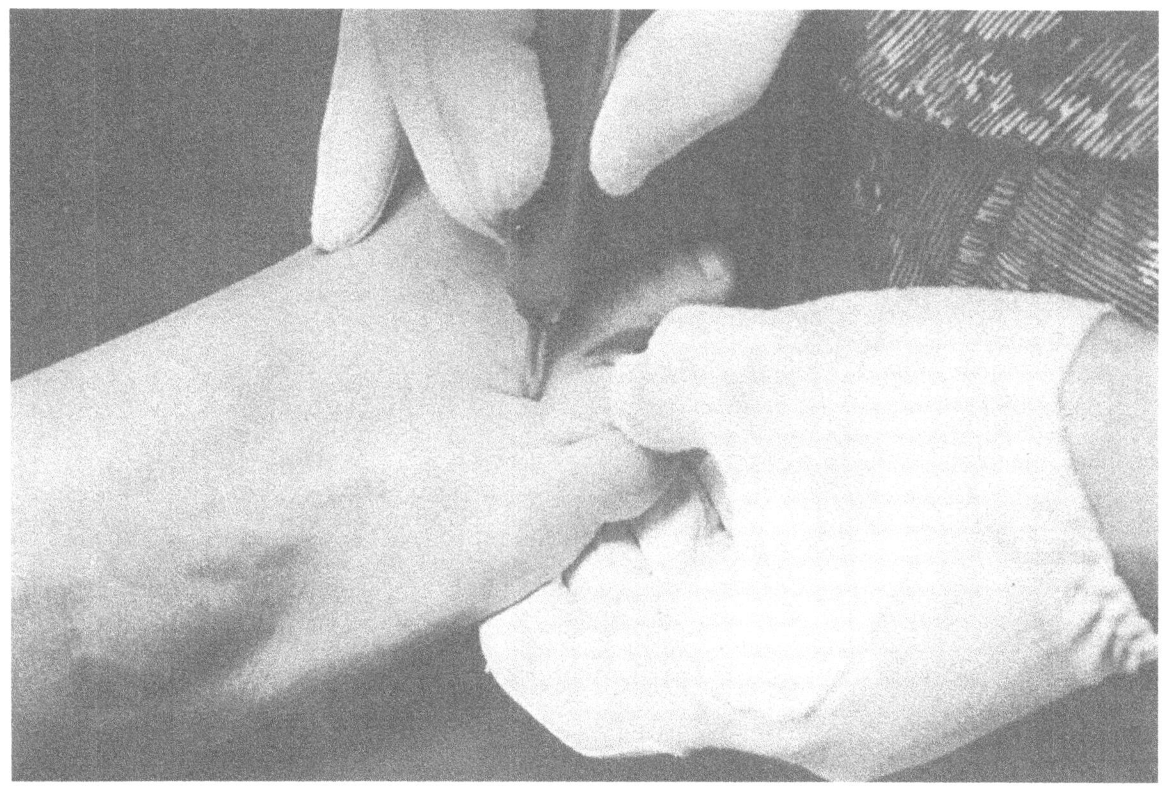

Fatty Degeneration

4. MP-3 — Organs and vessels in the head, brain, cerebral malacia, cerebral sclerosis.

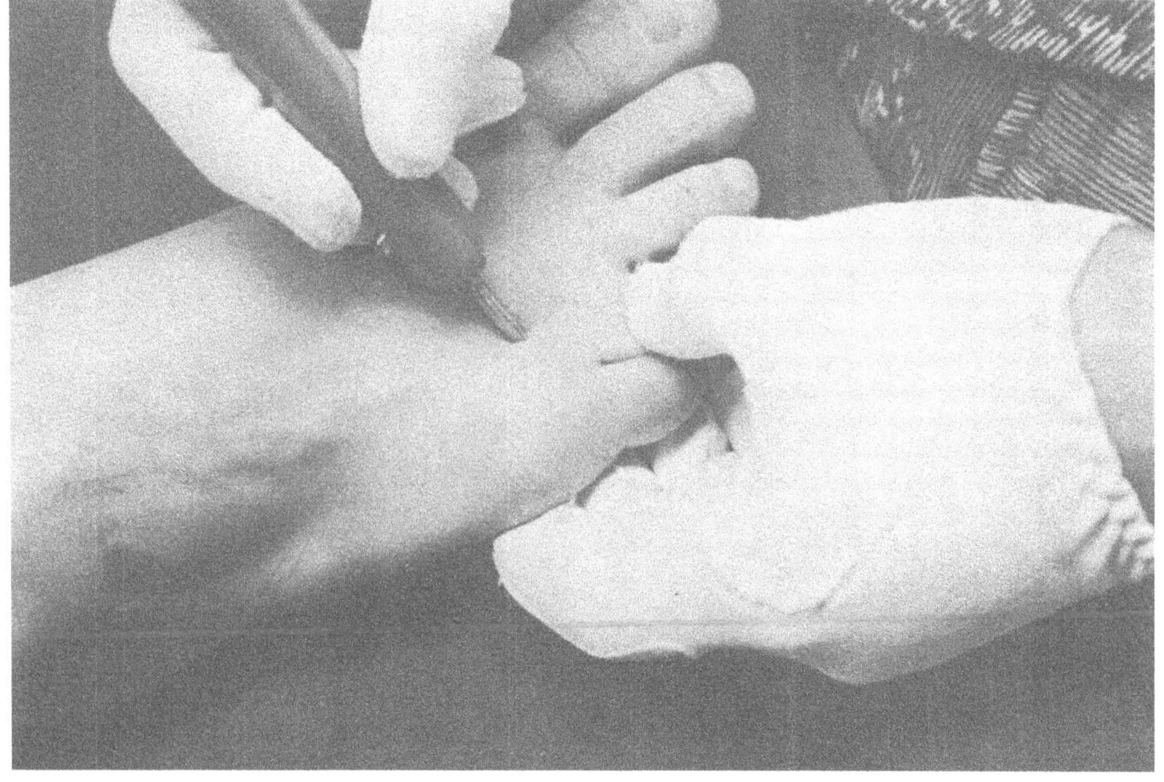

Gallbladder

Voll's *Illustrated Volume II, fig.* 13a, p. 34; fig. 13b, p. 35.

Functional disturbances in biliary system may affect the sleep centers in diencephalon and mesencephalon (falling asleep).

1. MP-44 — Ductus choledochus — right, ductus hepaticus communis — left.
2. MP-43c —Plexus hepaticus (right only).

RIGHT

3. *CMP — (compare with ID of liver).*
4. *MP-44a — Peritoneum.*
5. *MP-43 — Ductus cysticus.*
6. *MP-42 — Gallbladder (right toot).*
7. *MP-41 — Ductuli biliferi in the right liver lobe.*
8. *MP-39 — Bone marrow.*
9. *MP-34 — Muscles of lower extremities (lower back pain).*
10. *MP-29 — Hip joint, 3rd measurement point.*
11. *MP-20 — Sympathetic SMP.*
12. *MP-16 — Center for deep sleep (insomnia).*
13. *MP-17 — Formatio Reticularis.*
14. *MP-41 — Midbrain, mesencephalon, center of sleep and wake rhythm.*
15. *MP-8 — Tuber cinereum above ear on parietosquamous suture balanced by cranial ganglia.*
16. *MP-4 — Thalamus — speech.*

2. *CMP — (compare with ID of liver).*

LEFT

3. *MP-P — Peritoneum.*
4. MP-43 — Ductus hepaticus.
5. *MP-42 — Ductus hepaticus sinister.*
6. *MP-41 — Ductule biliferi in left liver lobe.*
7. *MP-42 — Hepatic duct.*

NOTES

Gallbladder

1. MP-44 — Ductus choledochus — right, ductus hepaticus communis — left.

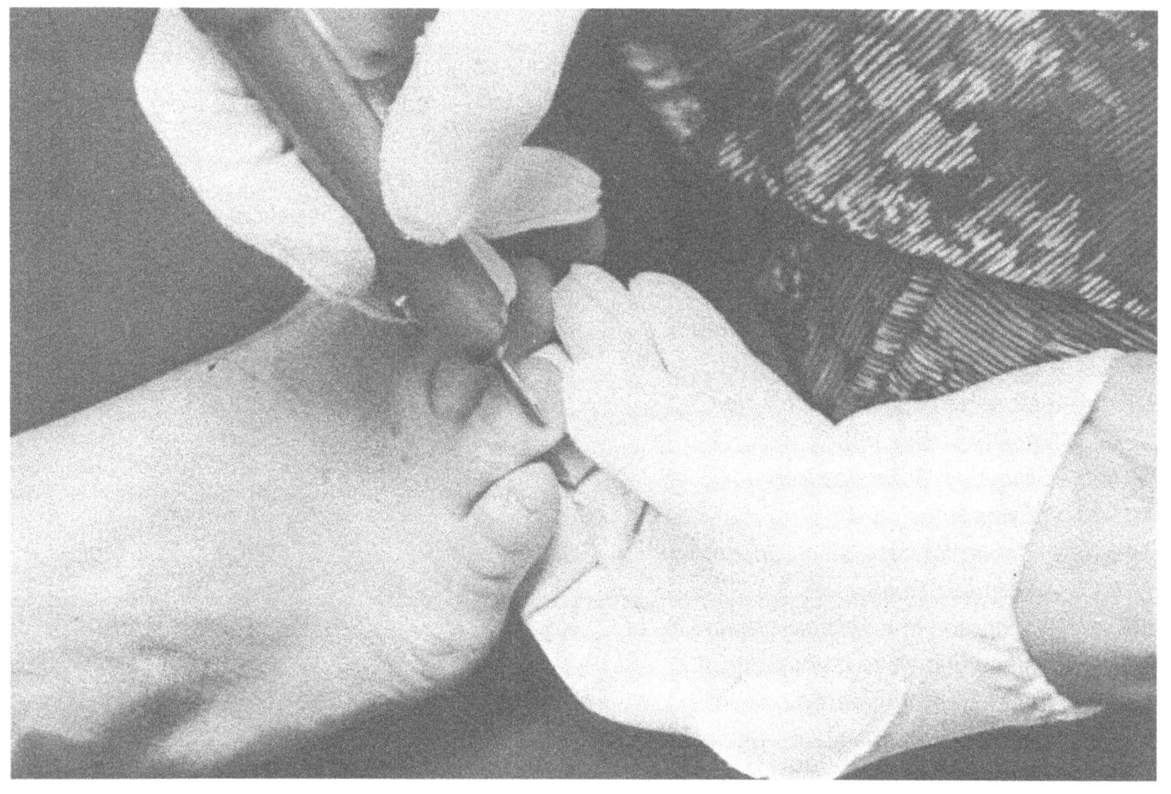

Gallbladder

3. *CMP — (compare with ID of liver).* Right. 2. *CMP — (compare with ID of liver).* Left.

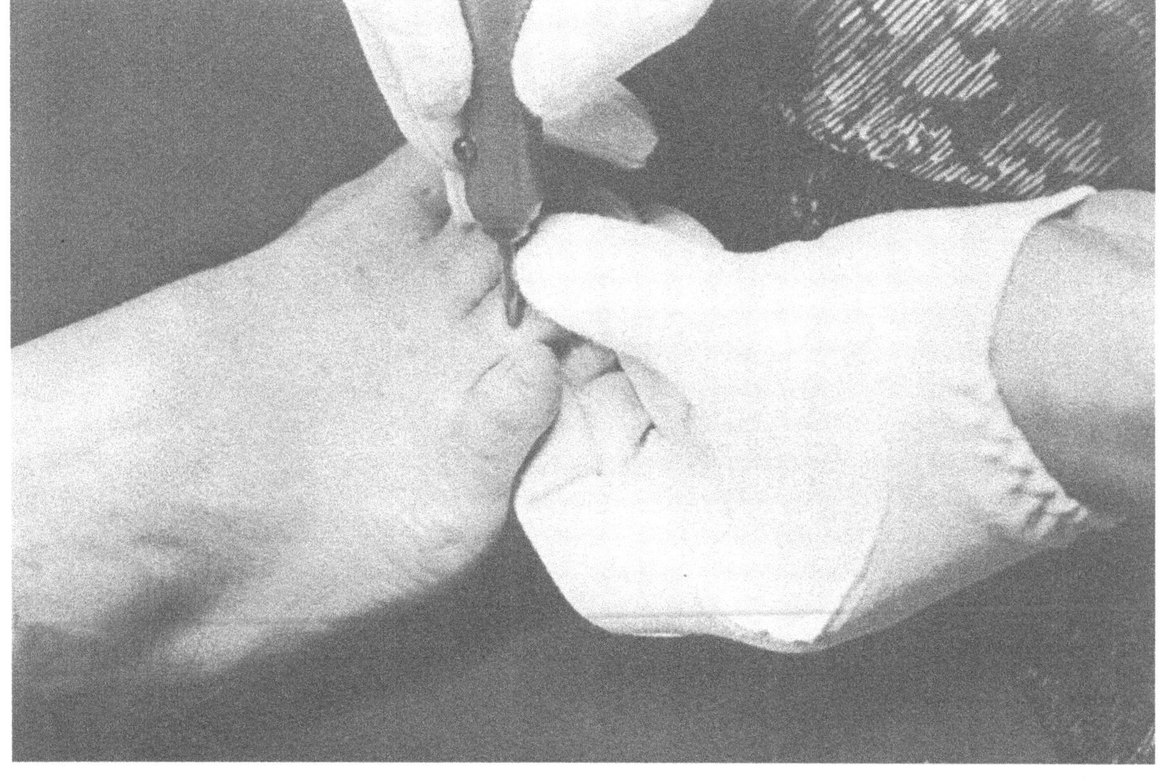

Kidney

Voll's *Illustrated Volume I*, illus. 14, p. 105.

May be influenced by lymphatic drainage of the ear, Ly 1 -1.

Closely associated with adrenal gland, check blood pressure on both sides of the arm.

1. MP-1 — Renal pelvis.
2. MP-Ki-1 a — Urethra, urinary congestion — hydronephrosis intermittent; cramping from urinary inability to urinate. Take blood pressure both sides. Colic complaints of unspecific origin. Measure also peritoneum of Ki from adhesions, shades, contusion.
3. MP-1-1 — Renal plexus.
4. CMP — Kidney.
5. MP-1 b — Suprarenal plexus (hypoglycemia point — according to Khoe).
6. MP-2 — Pyelorenal boundary layer (lymphatic swelling may indicate kidney stones).
7. MP-2a — Medulla of the straight canicili and collecting tubules.
8. MP-3 — Cortex of kidney.
9. MP-4a — Sphincter ani (right side).
10. MP-5 — Anal canal (hemorrhoids — right side).
11. MP-6 — Rectum (right side).
12. MP-10a — Medulla of adrenal gland.
13. MP-10b — Cortex of adrenal gland.

NOTES

Kidney

1. MP-1 —Renal pelvias

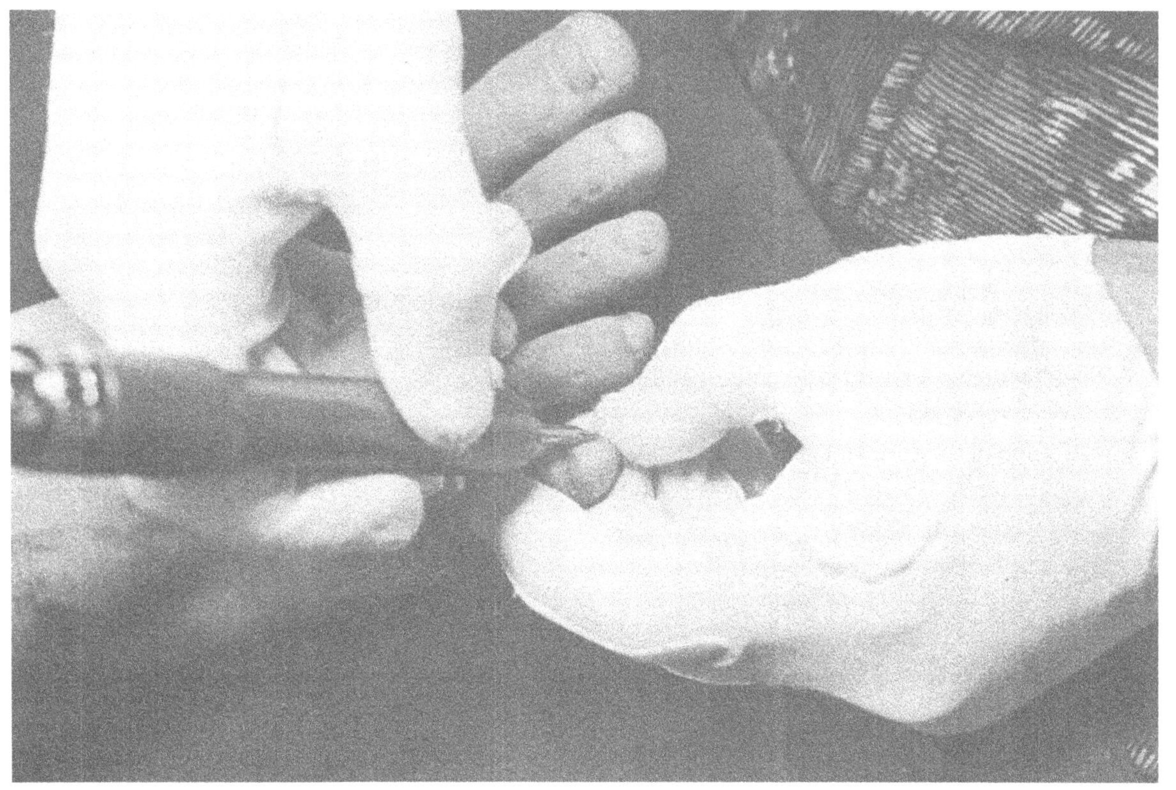

Kidney

2. MP-Ki-1a — Urethra, urinary congestion.

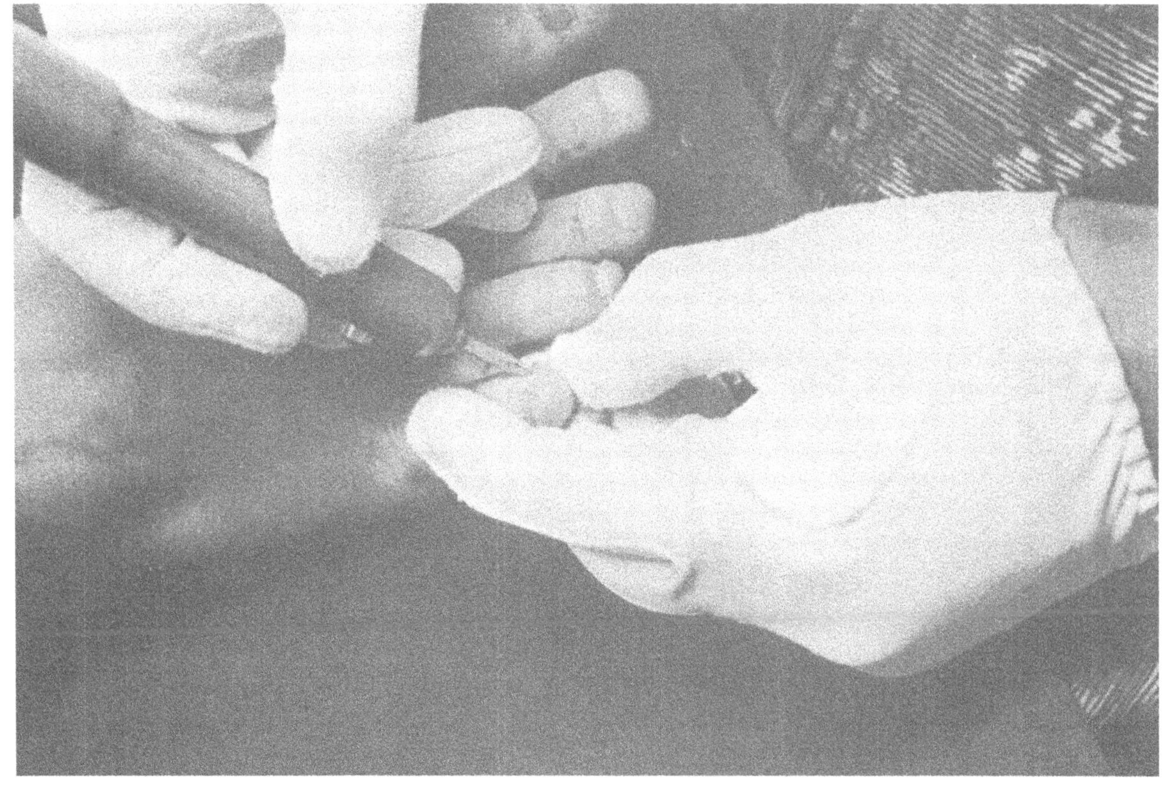

Kidney

3. MP-1-1 — Renal plexus.

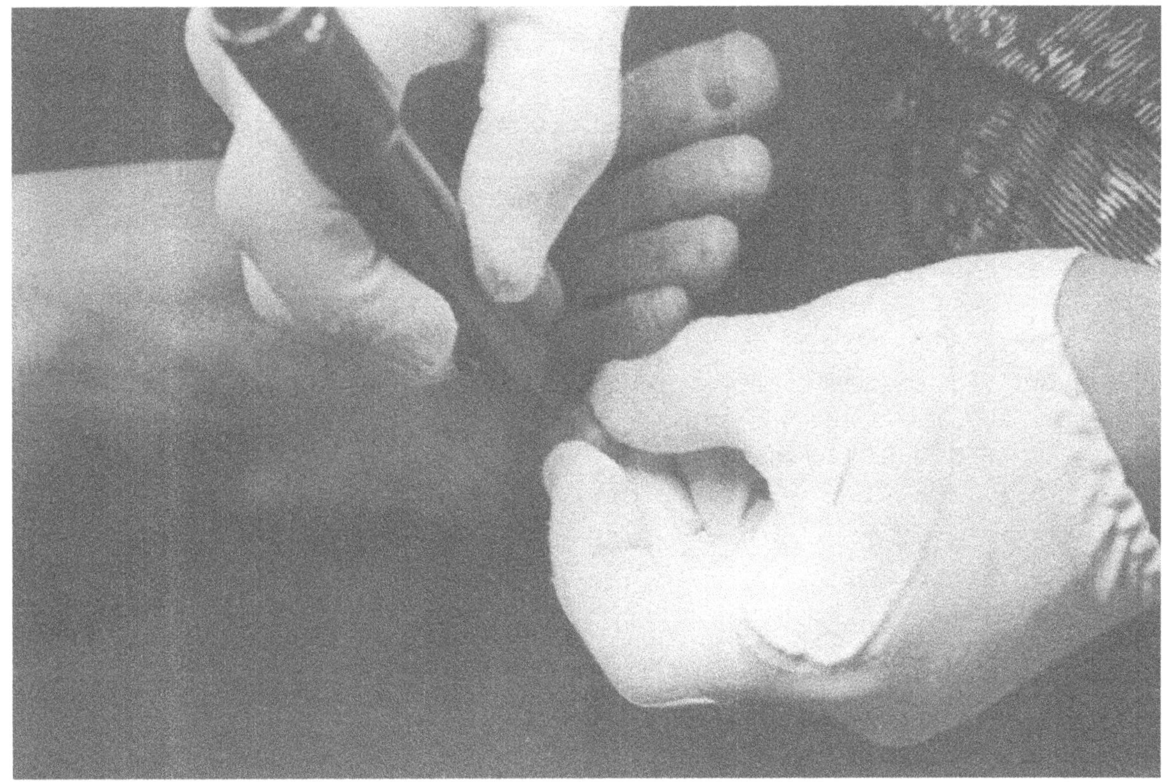

Kidney

4. CMP — Kidney.

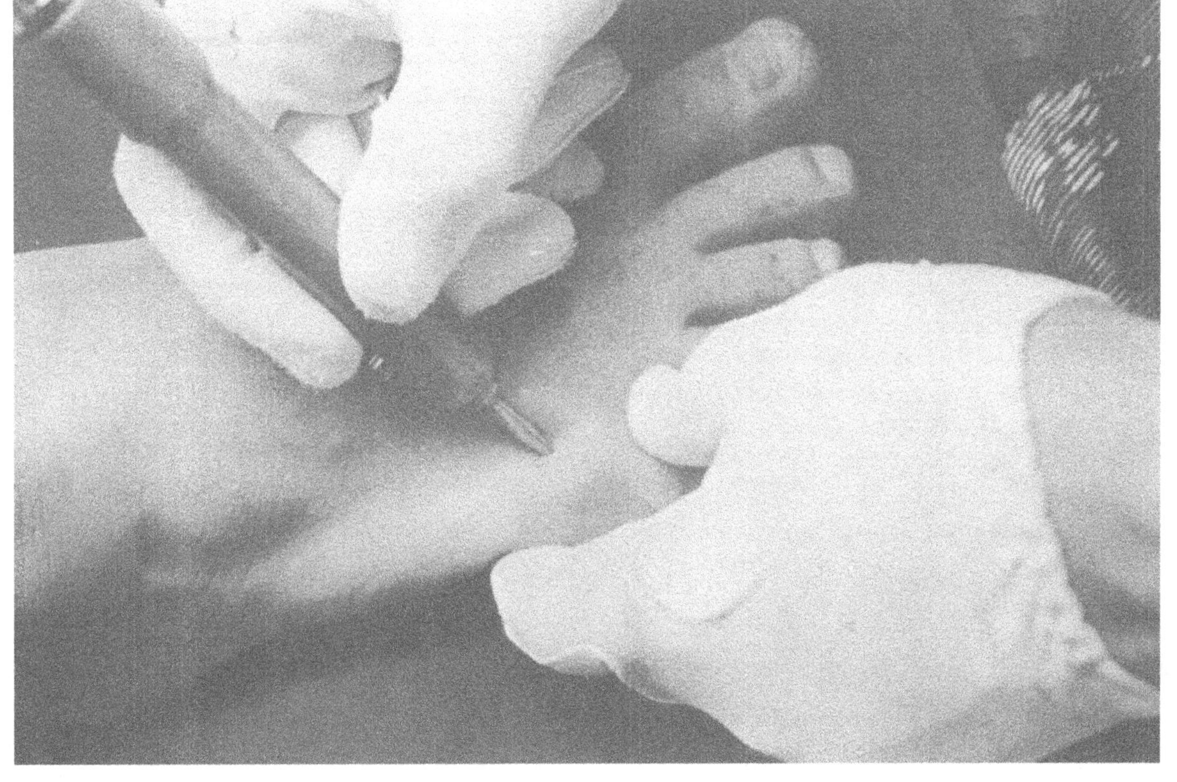

Urinary Bladder

Voll's *Illustrated Volume III,* figs. 9a, 9b, p. 121.

1. MP-67 — Body of the urinary bladder.
2. MP-66c — Bladder plexus.
3. CMP — Bladder.
4. MP-66 — Fundus cervix, sphincter of urinary bladder, collum and base of the urinary bladder.
5. MP-P — Peritoneum.
6. MP-65 — Summation point for reproductive organs for male and female:
    a. MP-49c — Seminal vesicle or pars intersitialis uteri.
    b. MP-50 — Prostate gland, lateral prostatic lobe; uterus (corpus uteri).
    c. MP-50-1 — Middle prostatic lobe.
    d. MP-50-2 — Prostatic sinus; female-portio vaginalis in uteri.
    e. MP-50a — Seminal hillock or broad ligament with parametria.
    f. MP-50b — Cowper's or Bartholini's gland.
    g. MP-51 — Penis or vagina.
    h. MP-51 a — Urethra, posterior portion.
7. MP-64 — Summation point for epididymis, spermatic cord in males, fallopian tubule in females:
    a. MP-49a — Epididymis or ostium abdominal tubae.
    b. MP-49b — Spermatic cord or ampulla tubae — occurs in late 50's, early 60's. Usually part of it. Commonly is pelvic neuralgia.
8. MP-63 — SMP lower hypogastric plexus.
9. MP-61 — Lumbar spine, sacrum, coccyx (lower back pain).
10. MP-60 — Nerves of the lower extremities.
11. MP-43 — Right side — caused by coxsackie virus for neuralgia of the back and shoulder (according to Khoe).
12. MP-35 — Preganglionic fibers of parasympathetics, sacral, medulla.
13. MP-34 — Pelvic plexus.

NOTES

14. MP-33 — Pelvic portion o,' sympathetic.
15. MP-32 — Sacrum, penis.
16. MP-29 — Thoracic vertebrae.
17. MP-28 — Bladder associated reflex (according to Khoe).
18. MP-27 — Small intestine associated reflex (ilio sacral joint according to Khoe).
19. MP-25 — Large intestine associated reflex (according to Khoe).
20. MP-24 — Abdominal part of sympathetic.
21. MP-23 — Kidney gland associated reflex (according to Khoe).
22. MP-22 — Adrenal gland associated reflex (according to Khoe).
23. MP-21 — Stomach associated reflex.
24. MP-20 — Spleen, pancreas associated reflex.
25. MP-19 — Gallbladder associated reflex.
26. MP-18 — Liver associated reflex.
27. MP-17 — Conception vessel associated reflex, MP for diaphragm left-hiatus hernia.
28. MP-16 — Governing vessel associated reflex, thoracic of sympathetic.
29. MP-15 — Heart associated reflex.
30. MP-14 — Circulation sex associated reflex.
31. MP-13 — Lung associated reflex (chronic cough).
32. MP-12 — Osseous system fractures of bones of all kinds, contusion, distortion.
33. MP-11 — Entire spine.
34. MP-10c — Inferior cervical ganglion.
35. MP-10b — Cervical medial ganglion VII.
36. MP-10a — Superior cervical ganglion.
37. MP-10 — Medulla Oblongata.
38. MP-9 — Pons (trigeminal neuralgia).
39. MP-2 — Frontal sinus — connected to LI-20, ethmoid cells by secondary vessel.
40. MP-2a — Brain stem.

NOTES

Urinary Bladder

1. MP-67 — Body of the urinary bladder.

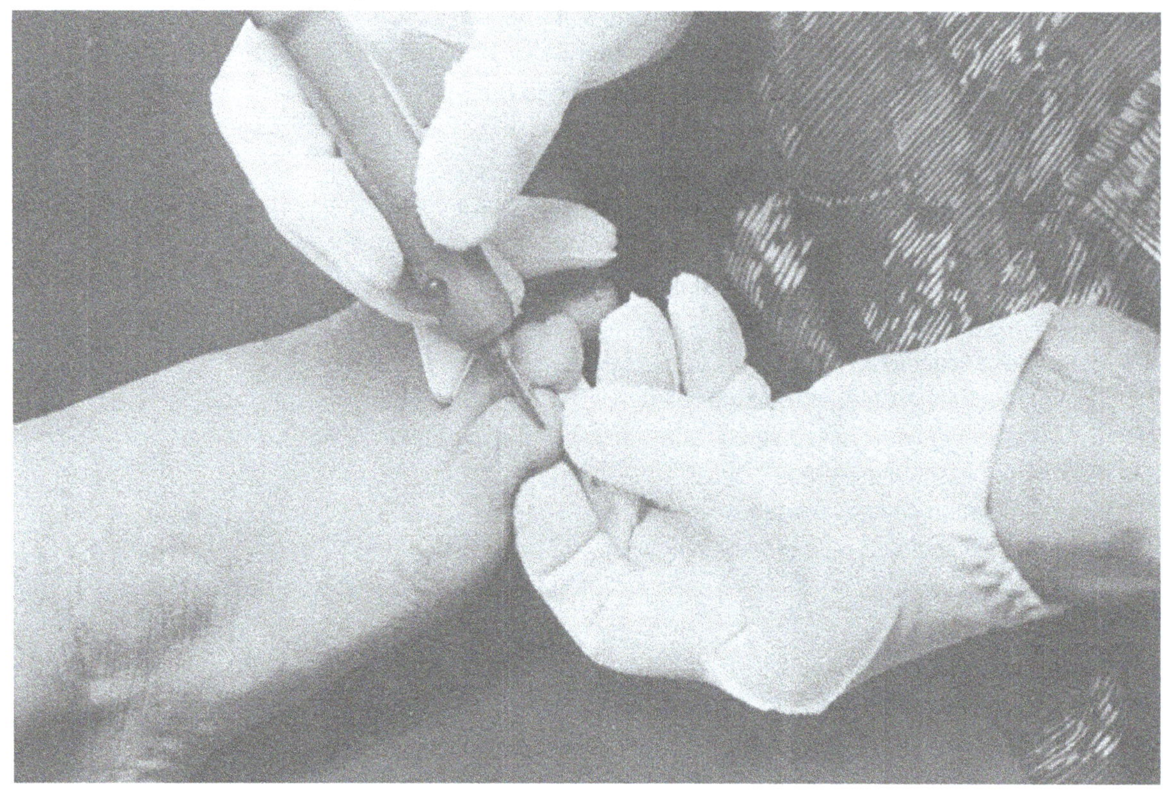

Urinary Bladder

3. CMP — Bladder.

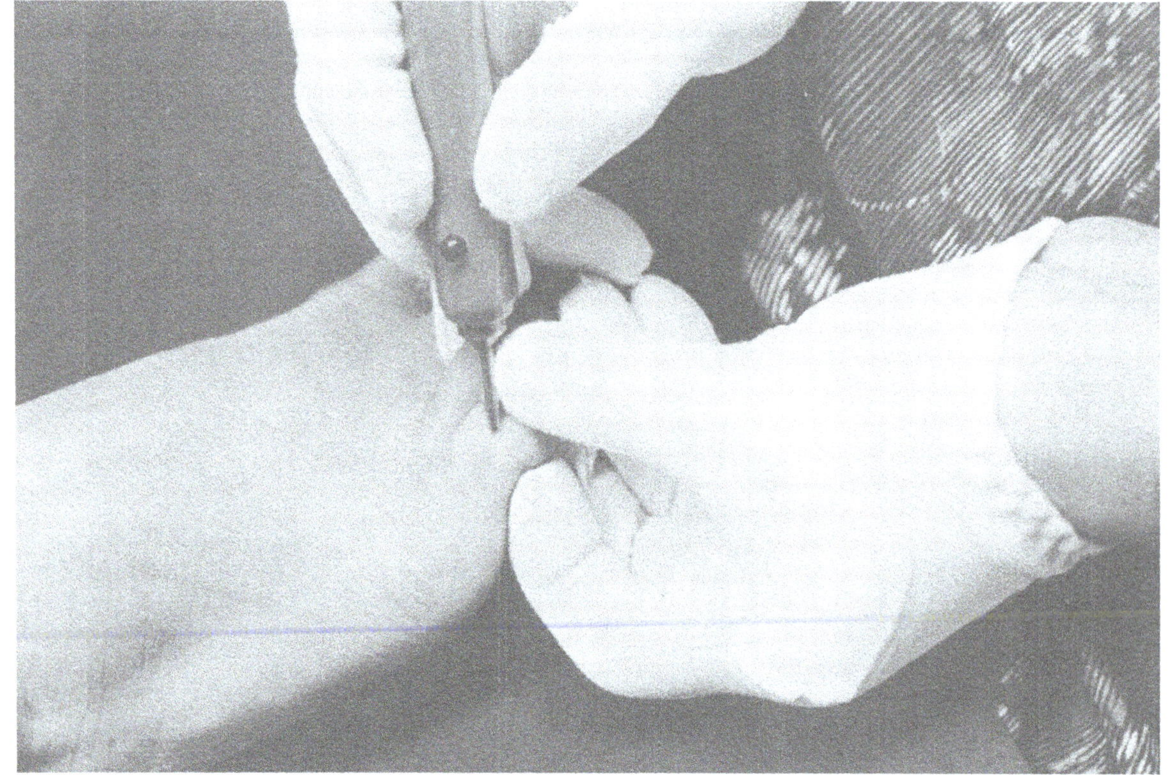

Urinary Bladder

6. MP-65 — Summation point for reproductive organs for male and female.

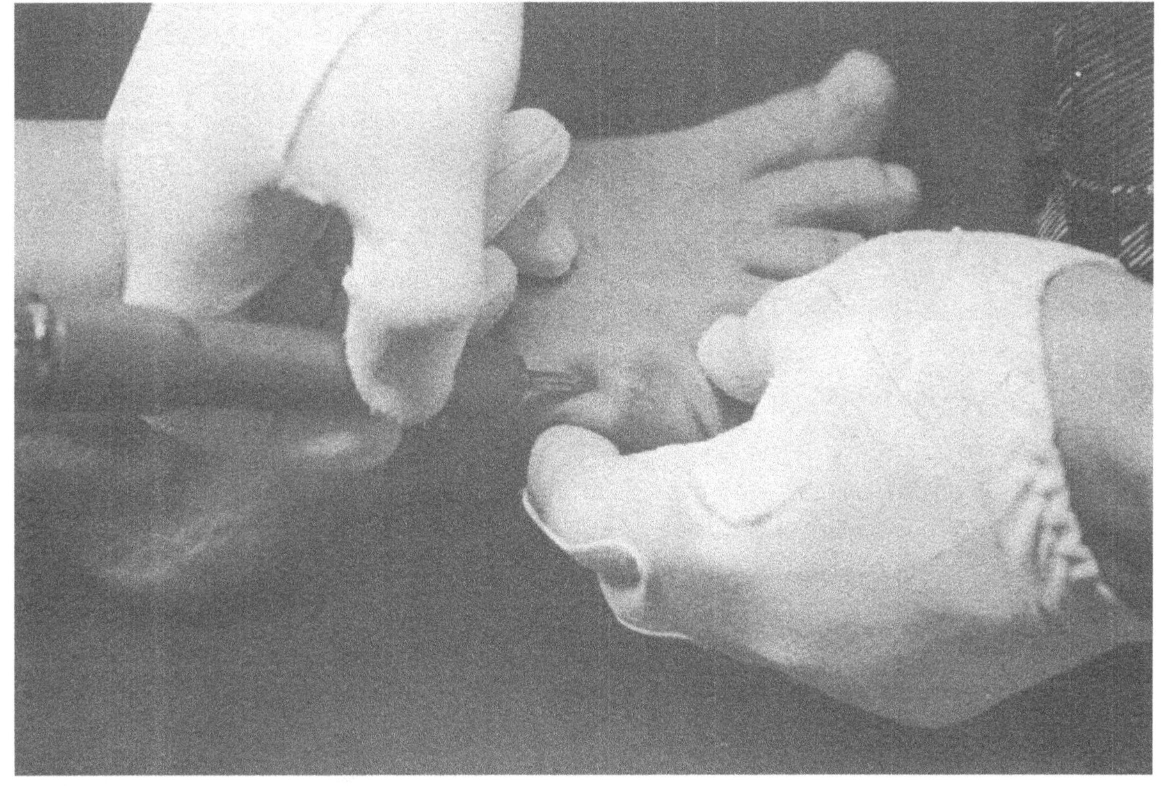

NOTES

BODY ELECTRO-ACUPUNCTURE POINTS ACCORDING TO VOLL

Conception Vessel

1. *MP-24 — Lower jaw section (1st bicuspid to lower bicuspid).*
2. *MP-23c — Pharyngeal tonsil.*
3. *MP-21 — Larynx.*
4. *MP-17 — Alarm point (circulation-sex) (pericardium) (precordial pain).*
5. *MP-15, 17, 21 — Intercostal.*
6. *MP-14 — Alarm point — heart.*
7. *MP-12 — Alarm point — stomach (check also C\J-12 St. 21 for stomach pain).*
8. *MP-7 — Scrotum pain.*
9. *MP-5 — Alarm point TW.*
10. *MP-4 — Alarm point SI.*
11. *MP-3 — Alarm point — bladder (uterus pain).*

Governing Vessel

1. *MP-25 — Upper anterior jaw MP — 1st bicuspid to 1st bicuspid.*
2. *MP-23-1 — CMP — cerebrum (stroke, headaches).*
3. MP-23-2 — *Limbic point control.*
4. *MP-23 — Hippocampus, hairline (for memory).*
5. *MP-23a — Nasal cavity.*
6. *MP-22 — MP Gyrus cinguli.*
7. *MP-22, 23 — Swallowing pain (check also Voll St-10).*
8. *MP-21 — Corpus amygdaloideum.*
9. *MP-20 — Visual point (jet lag, headaches, vertigo, neurasthenia).*
10. *MP-19 — MP-little brain, anterior lobe (headaches, dizziness, stiff neck, reflex point of anterior cerebellum. Also balancing problem of multiple sclerosis, lateral sclerosis and stroke).*
11. *MP-19a — Posterior lobe, cerebellum.*
12. *MP-19b — Archicerebellum.*
13. *MP-16, 28 — SMP — neck portion of the sympathetics (tor nape pain).*
14. *MP-15 — Chronic headaches.*
15. *MP-14-2 — Spinal marrow.*
16. *MP-14 — For high fever (thoracic I).*
17. *MP-13 — Spinal marrow — medulla of spinal cord.*
18. *MP-9, 11 — Intercostal pain.*

NOTES

Yin and Yang Principle of Opposites

Yin and Yang on the Organ Clock

Oriental philosophy teaches that there are two opposing energies necessary to life and health — the Yin and the Yang. The balance between these forces is influenced by time, weather, seasons and occurrences in nature. Disease results from an imbalance between the Yin and the Yang.

The Yin is a name given to the force which causes expansion. Drugs (including alcohol) for example, tend to cause physiological and mental expansion. In other words, Yin dissipates. Elements which tend to make us dizzy or light-headed when taken as food or medicine are Yin. It takes a binding force (yang) to balance the great expansion created by Yin. From this difficulty in maintaining equilibrium, all kinds of sickness arise.

Yang represents energy.

The Yin on the organ clock represents the circulatory system, the heart, the sexual, spleen, lung, kidney and liver organs. These solid organs store energy produced by the Yang. They also distribute energy. Yin expands, sedates and is inert. In pulse diagnosis, the Yin is the deep pulse.

The Yang tends to make things contract, to be dense and heavy. When the Yang is dominant, a given element will contract. Yang does not cause dizziness as Yin does. Salt, soy sauce, ginseng, etc., are rather effective in relieving dizziness. However, they should not be taken in excess as they will produce the opposite effect.

The Yang on the organ clock represents the bladder, large intestine, gallbladder, stomach, small intestine, and triple warmer. The Yang feeds and excretes and is the hollow organ, giving a superficial pulse meridian in pulse diagnosis.

NOTES

All organs are in pairs. As the general circulation of energy flows through the meridian, the polarity changes from Yin to Yang or Yang to Yin — from meridian to meridian. The coupling point is at the end of one meridian and the beginning of the next. The following are divided equally into the Yin and the Yang as related to the teeth. According to Voll, the following meridians are influenced by certain teeth and influence certain organs:

YIN MERIDIANS	YANG MERIDIANS	TEETH
Kidney	Bladder	Central and lateral, upper and lower
Lung	Large intestine	Upper 1st bicuspid, lower 1st molar — lung Upper 2nd bicuspid, lower 2nd molar — large intestine
Liver	Gallbladder	Cuspid, upper and lower — both
Pancreas (right side)	Stomach	Upper 1st molar, lower 1st bicuspid — pancreas-spleen
Spleen (left side)		Upper 2nd molar, lower 2nd bicuspid — stomach
Heart	Small intestine	3rd molar, upper and lower
Circulatory system/sexual organs	Triple warmer	3rd molar, upper and lower
Refer to ODONTON on the ORGAN TISSUE CHART for more information.		

The Balancing of Yin and Yang

Each meridian has a two hour peak energy time and 12 hours later, a two hour low energy time. If a mild stimulus such as a tonification or sedation is applied to the meridian, only that meridian is affected. If the stimulus is intense on that meridian, then the opposite meridian is affected (sedated). Since one organ of the pair is Yang and the other is Yin, there is a balancing effect. Thus it is important to treat both organs and keep them balanced.

If there is a toothache on the anterior central and lateral teeth, you should suspect an overabundance of energy on the bladder and kidney meridians where the pain would be from 3 to 7 P.M. with generalized tiring on the upper part of the body in the lung and large intestine meridians from 3 to 7 A.M. (12 hours away from the toothache). Therefore, by sedating the toothache at the time of pain (3 to 7 A.M.) by treating the tooth with a mild stimulus, you can control the high created by that tooth on that meridian only.

If a patient has a headache at a certain time — for example, 1 to 3 P.M. — on the organ clock, you should suspect that he has an excess of energy in the small intestine and a low energy at 1 to 3 A.M. which is the liver. Sedation at 1 to 3 P.M. will relieve the headache and bring the energy down. This is using a mild stimulus and will only affect that meridian of maximum time. If the stimulus is intense, the opposite meridian, 12 hours later, will have the opposite effect of sedation.

You will also notice that a person who has had toothache pain relieved will also have an energy increase several hours later.

The healing process can be accomplished by energizing or sedating, using low frequency oscillating current with the Dermatron electro-acupuncture instruments on the meridian control points of the foot and hand as found in classical acupuncture and by Voll. Another alternative is using the footplates to energize and balance with low alternating electric current on the four quadrants of the body. In this way, the body will circulate and adjust its own deficiencies and surpluses of energy. Consequently, an equilibrium of energy will be produced among the meridians.

ORGAN CLOCK

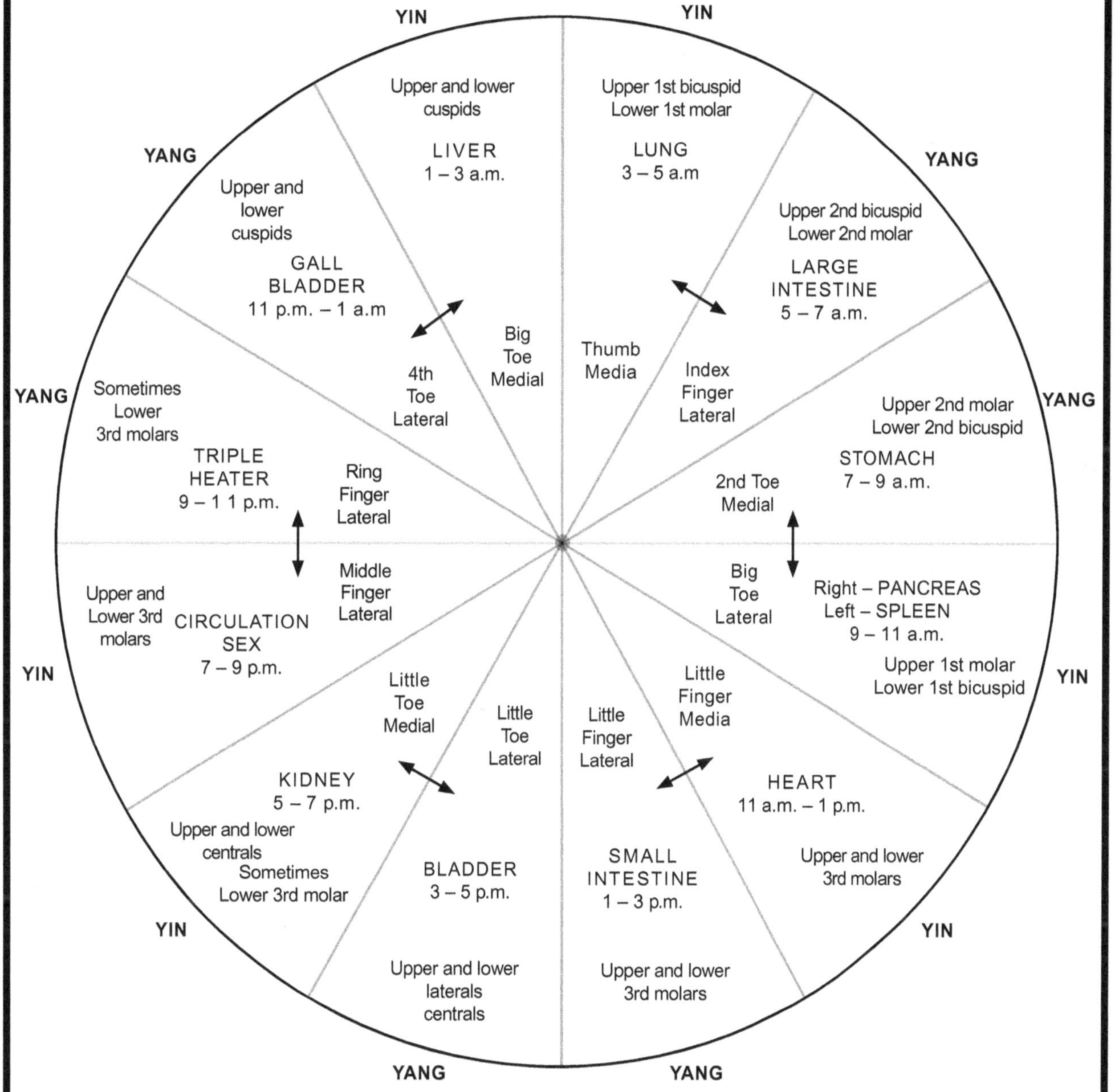

YIN
YIN
YANG
YANG
YANG
YANG
YIN
YIN
YIN
YIN
YANG
YANG
Upper and lower cuspids
LIVER
1 – 3 a.m.
Big Toe Medial
Upper 1st bicuspid
Lower 1st molar
LUNG
3 – 5 a.m
Thumb Media
Upper 2nd bicuspid
Lower 2nd molar
LARGE INTESTINE
5 – 7 a.m.
Index Finger Lateral
Upper 2nd molar
Lower 2nd bicuspid
STOMACH
7 – 9 a.m.
2nd Toe Medial
Big Toe Lateral
Right – PANCREAS
Left – SPLEEN
9 – 11 a.m.
Upper 1st molar
Lower 1st bicuspid
Little Finger Media
HEART
11 a.m. – 1 p.m.
Upper and lower 3rd molars
Little Finger Lateral
SMALL INTESTINE
1 – 3 p.m.
Upper and lower 3rd molars
Little Toe Lateral
BLADDER
3 – 5 p.m.
Upper and lower laterals centrals
Little Toe Medial
KIDNEY
5 – 7 p.m.
Upper and lower centrals
Sometimes Lower 3rd molar
Middle Finger Lateral
Upper and Lower 3rd molars
CIRCULATION SEX
7 – 9 p.m.
Ring Finger Lateral
Sometimes Lower 3rd molars
TRIPLE HEATER
9 – 1 1 p.m.
4th Toe Lateral
Upper and lower cuspids
GALL BLADDER
11 p.m. – 1 a.m

The following is how the Yang and the Yin work in the disease process:

YANG	YIN
ACUTE	CHRONIC
FEVER	SUBNORMAL TEMPERATURE
FEELS HOT	FEELS COLD
DRY	MOIST
POWERFUL	WEAK
SPREADING	DOMINANT
ACTIVE	NON-ACTIVE

ENERGETIC REACTIONS BETWEEN THE ODONTONS AND THE ORGANS AND TISSUE SYSTEMS

Odonton Numbering System 1-8

Five Ventilated Sinuses Related to the Organs and Teeth

1. Frontal sinus — UBL-2, upper and lower centrals and laterals.
2. Sphenoid sinus, between LI-20 and UBL-1 on the secondary vessel at the end of the sutura nasomaxillaries in the transition zone of the osseous and the cartilage portion of the nose; upper and lower centrals, lateral and cuspids.
3. Ethmoid cells LI-20; upper 1st and 2nd bicuspids, lower 1st and 2nd molars.
4. Maxillary sinus St-5; upper 1st and 2nd molars, lower 1st and 2nd bicuspids.
5. Middle ear TW-17, internal ear TW-18.

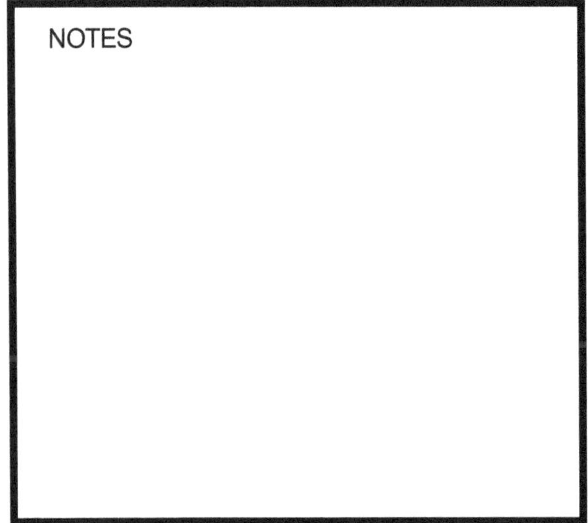

In general:

1. The lower canine irritates the anterior portion of the eye, conjunctiva and vitreous body.
2. The upper canine irritates posterior portion of the eye, retina, choriodea and retrobulbar portion of the optic nerve.
3. The lower 8 odonton affects the external and middle ear irritation.
4. The upper 8 odonton influences the internal ear including organs of balance and acoustics, intermittent occurring tinnitus and disturbances in balance such as dizziness which tend to improve gradually until the next toxic attack aggravates the situation. These are all indications of odontogenic etiology.

The odontogenic irritation of one of the paranasal sinuses can have two effects:

1. Predisposition to a unilateral catarrh (mild inflammation of the mucous membrane) when a focus is present on one side only.
2. In refractory (resistant to treatment) processes otherwise responding easily to therapy.

The foci of infection from the odontons can cause serious sinusitis which in turn may affect the vertebrae spine and spinal marrow. There is a direct correlation between cervical vertebrae 1 and 2 to a tooth irritation. Likewise, .the third and fourth cervical vertebrae indicates a paranasal inus irritation. Sinusitis can also have a reverse reaction creating sensitivity to the teeth.

Frontal sinusitis can manifest itself as a headache. The patient may also experience pain in the vertebrae spine L2, L3, S2, S3, S5 and coccyx. The spinal marrow may be affected in the SL2, SL3 lower portion of the plexus lumbalis, SS3, SS4, SS5 plexus pudendus coccygeus and plexus coccygeus.

Maxillary sinusitis, ethmoid cells, sphenoid, middle ear and the internal ear may also affect the vertebrae and the spinal marrow. (Refer to the dental chart.)

Special attention should be given to the sphenoidal sinus which is situated near the cavernous sinus. Bacteria in the sphenoid sinus can affect the cavernous sinus and the nerves and arteries which pass through it. The abducens, oculomotor, trochlear and opthalmic nerves (in addition to the internal carotid artery which is encircled by the sympathetic plexus caroticus internus) may be affected by an inflammation of the sphenoid sinus.

This may ultimately lead to an arterial hypertensive patient. The carotid artery is of great importance for the lymph system. This is where the material exchange between the liquor of the nerve sheaths of the mentioned cranial nerves and the beginning lymph vessels of the paranasal sinuses occurs; that is, the detoxification of the liquor in the subarachnoidal space and meninges. Inflammations of the sphenoidal sinus may also be caused by an inflammation in the terminal colon and its surroundings and cause further irritations to the vertebrae spine. (Refer to dental chart.)

Odontons Relation to the Tonsils

The tonsils likewise can also be irritated by the odontons and vice versa. Tenderness on the 3rd and 4th cervical is an indication of a focated or inflamed tonsil. Inflamed tonsils may affect organs, paranasal sinuses, sense organs, odontons, vertebrae spine, spinal marrow, joints and other tonsils. (Refer to dental chart.) The tonsils act like lymph glands. There are five tonsils, not including the appendix which some consider a small intestine tonsil. The five tonsils corresponding to the odontons are as follows:

1. Pharyngeal tonsils, upper and lower anterior central and laterals.
2. Palatine tonsils, upper and lower 1st and 2nd molar, upper 1st and 2nd bicuspids.
3. Laryngeal tonsils, lower 1st and 2nd bicuspids, upper 1st and 2nd molars.
4. Lingual tonsils, upper and lower wisdom teeth.
5. Tubal tonsils.

In the past, it was routine to remove the palatine tonsils in infants. This led to the belief by some patients that their tonsils were no longer present. However, little did they realize that they still have four other paired tonsils located in their head area. If there is an indicator drop reading on the palatine tonsil measurement point after that tonsil was removed by surgery, then remnants of that tonsil remain which can be the source of infection.

Besides having an effect on the odontons, the tonsils may affect other organs and tissues:

1. The pharyngeal tonsil CV-23c, disturbs the kidney and genito-urinary.
2. Palatine tonsils Lu-1, disturb the liver and gallbladder.
3. Tubal tonsils Lu-1 a, disturb the lung and large intestine.
4. Lingual tonsils St-3a, disturb the heart and small intestine.
5. Both the tubal and palatine tonsils disturb the appendix of small children.

When measuring the tonsillar ring and readings drop from 88 to 82, there is a typical focal value. Tonsillar focal disturbances can play an important role in adolescent and pre-teen children or in normalizing the ID to a stable value. If the tonsil point is balanced to 50, and if the corresponding tooth measurement point drops more than 10 units, the tonsils should be considered one of the foci of infection because children do not have teeth foci.

Odonton Relation to the Vertebrae

Tenderness in the 1st and 2nd cervical (atlas and axis) indicates a focus of irritation which may originate from the teeth. Palpate lightly along the transverse axis of the spine. A tender spot will usually show red. This indicates that the vertebrae is subluxated. (Refer to the dental chart.) Match the vertebrae with the corresponding tooth. Test the spot with the Dermatron to see if the vertebrae is inflamed, irritated or degenerative. Sedate to 50 the odonton Ly-MP-2 and see if the vertebrae value is reduced to 50. If it is, the tooth is the foci of infection. One odontogenic focus always irritates 2 or 3 successive vertebrae. An odontogenic focus causing a secondary tonsillogenic irritation always irritates simultaneously the 1, 2, 3 and 4 cervical vertebraes.

The following odontons can affect the following vertebraes:

1. C1, 2 ... irritated by all odontons.
2. C3, 04 . .. irritated by all tonsils of the tonsillar lymphatic ring. Usually the tonsillogenic foci are secondarily caused by the odontogenic foci.
3. C5, 06, 07 . . . lower 6, 7, upper 4, 5.
4. T1, T2 . . . all 8th odontons, wisdom teeth.
5. T3, T4 . . . lower 6, 7, upper 4, 5.
6. T5, T6, T7 . . . all wisdom teeth.
7. T8, T9, T10 . . . all cuspids.
8. T11, T12, L1 . . . lower 4, 5, upper 5, 6.
9. L2, L3 . . . all centrals and laterals.
10. L4, L5 . . . lower 6, 7, upper 4, 5.
11. S1, S2 . .. all wisdom teeth.
12. S3, S4, S5 and coccyx ... all centrals and laterals.

Differential diagnosis, using the roller electrodes of the Dermatron, are as follows:

1. The roller with the black plug is placed on the spine.
2. The other electrode (red) stylus at a distance of 3 finger breadth with water is used to record the values of the focated area. Compare the reading with a non-focated area adjacent to the spine.

Odonton Relation to the Spinal Segments and Dermatomes

Irritation from the teeth can also cause carbuncles, furuncles and rash around the body. Again, if a rash, carbuncles or furuncles are located in cervical 1 and 2, it can be related to the teeth. The teeth foci is usually differentiated from other fields of disturbance by being unilateral and involving one or two teeth related to one or two segments. If the tonsils or the parasinuses are involved, then cervicals 1 to 4 are involved. Infections to the sinuses, such as the sphenoid and cavernous, may complicate the diagnosis, especially that of smallpox which may be a fungating and multiple combining spore growth. Corresponding movements in the knee, upper extremities and lower extremities may be painful and may give clues to a disturbed segment of the spinal marrow.

Disturbances in the movement of the shoulder and upper arm may be due to odontogenic and tonsillogenic irritations, particularly the lower odontons 6, 7 and the upper odontons 4, 5. Disturbances in the movement of the lower arm and the hand can only be linked to the irritations originating in the lower odontons 6, 7 and to the upper odontons 4, 5. All coordinated movements of the feet and toes, thumbs and fingers may be irritated by the wisdom odonton only. Fibryotic scar adhesions may alter these movements and be the foci of infection itself.

Refer to the dental and dermatomes charts to analyze any dysfunction or disease when performing a posture analysis examination. With this information and the medical history, the doctor is able to test these symptoms with the Dermatron instruments.

Odontogenic Irritations on Muscles

Muscle groups can be irritated by various causes. Differential diagnosis must be made between muscular, articular and neural pains. Organs and their pairs may influence the function of muscle groups as evident in kinesiology. Diseases also must be considered. It is therefore important to be able to recognize the causes and not only the symptoms.

Muscles of the trunk are irritated by 12 odontons on one side, teeth 3-8 — cuspids to wisdom teeth, upper and lower. Muscles of the upper extremity are irritated by 3 odontons on one side — upper and lower molars. Muscles of the lower extremity are irritated by 10 odontons on one side — upper and lower odontons 1, 2, 8 odontons and the lower 6, 7 as well as the upper odontons 4, 5.

A paper presented by Khoe in the American Journal of Acupuncture, Vol. 6, No. 1, January-March, 1978 illustrates the relation of the muscles, related organs, meridians and alarm points.

This therapy is explained below:

1. Palpate the muscles until the painful muscle is located. Also determine the muscle restriction, if any is observed.
2. Compare this muscle with the organ and its meridian. A test with the EAV meter will reveal an indicator drop signifying a disturbance of that meridian. These tender acupuncture points can be injected bilaterally with B-12 injections to form a small wheel. If the pain is relieved, then the cause is found. Ultrasound therapy can be used instead of needles. EAV therapy can also be used under sedation therapy in balancing the inflamed measurement point to 50.
3. The associated point is then located. (Refer to associated points in EAV Dental Chart.) Insertion of B-12, ultrasound or EAV is again used to sedate the pain.
4. Then the related alarm point is located and treated as above.
5. The patient must strictly adhere to a diet free of red meat, refined sugars, chemical additives, preservatives, colorings, emulsifiers and stabilizers.

The EAV measurement point for muscles of the leg is GBL-MP-34, located on the lateral side of the knee while the measurement point of the muscles of the arm is SI-MP-9 on the medial upper portion of the arm.

Odontogenic Irritation on the Endocrine Glands

The endocrine glands can be affected by the odontons and vice versa. Most of the endocrine glands (or triple warmer meridian) are related to the upper teeth with the exception of the adrenal gland.

The following associations are as follows:

1. Pineal gland . . . UB-8 and upper and 2 odontons
2. Adrenal gland . . . UB-22 or TW-1, lower 1 and 2 odontons
3. Pituitary gland . . . GBL-20a, center mediate lobe — upper 3 odonton — cuspid
4. Pituitary gland . . . GBL-12, posterior lobe, upper 4 odonton
5. Thymus gland .. . St-11, upper 5 odonton
6. Thyroid gland . . . St-10, upper 6 odonton
7. Parathyroid gland . . . St-9, upper 7 odonton
8. Anterior pituitary lobe . . . GBL-21, SI-15, TW-16, upper 8 odonton
9. Gonad . . . St-31, LI-11, Sp-Pa-11, lower cuspids

The endocrine adrenal gland can be irritated by odontons 1-2 in the lower jaw while all odontons may irritate the head and neck area.

Oral focal infections can result often in the painful disturbances of the thyroid. This symptom is most often seen in tonsillogenic foci. In contrast, an odontogenic focal irritation results in dystyreosis, that is, the intermittent changes in hyper and hypofunctions.

When one mammary breast has been unequal in size to the other for years, an odontogenic irritation of the upper 5th tooth (thymus) and the lower 5th tooth (lymphatic system) is excluded. An equal formation of the mammary gland should be noted. There seems to be a smaller right breast in 30% of the women because of exercise of the pectoralis muscle in right-handed individuals. Irritations caused by these teeth always result in a lymphatic swelling which occurs suddenly. In contrast to this, formation of nodules in the mammary gland is caused by an odontogenic irritation of the lower 4, 5 and upper 6, 7 and occasionally also of the upper 5th odonton.

When an otogenic irritation is caused by the upper incisors, a temporary oliguria may result after a toxic attack because of the overproduction of aduretin. The pineal gland cannot counterbalance the aduretin of the posterior pituitary lobe.

Odontogenic irritation of the upper 4th tooth may cause a prolonged period of constipation resistant to purgative because of the lack of oxytocin. It also can cause the lack of contractive hormones of the posterior pituitary lobe to set on the muscles of the uterus. Amenorrhoea may occur from an upper impacted tooth #8.

An odontogenic irritation of the lower 1, 2 can cause a hyper and hypofunction symptom of the adrenal glands to be disguised and intensify corresponding symptoms based on this weakness. See if there is an inflamed gingivae around the lower 1 and 2 teeth. Hypotonia not responsive to circulatory medications is most often caused by the adrenal gland.

Female hormones (progesterone) often can cause a secretory phase in the menstruation cycle. Malfunctions of the ovaries caused by the foci of the lower 3, 4 odontons may result in disturbances of the period such as oligomenorrhoea (insufficient menstrual flow), hemorrhagia and rhythmic disturbances of the period.

In treating the syndrome of impotency associated with necrospermia, azoospermia or oliospermia, examine the lower 3, 4 odontons.

Odontogenic Irritations and their Neural Effects

Every focus irritates hypothalmus on the same side, 82 to 88 without an ID. The hypothalmus value of the side of the focus shows a higher value compared with the other side:

1. Dysregulation of the autonomic centers in the brain stem in the medulla oblongata.
2. Dysregulation of the autonomic cervical ganglia of the parasympathetic.
3. Cerebral irritations of the thymopsyche and limbic system.
4. Neural irritations to the cranial system.

The upper wisdom teeth can affect the limbic system (sexual and emotional points) and the central nervous system. The lower wisdom teeth affect the peripheral nervous system.

Odontogenic Irritations to the Intercostal Nerves

Intercostal nerves (ICN) of the thoracic segments of the spinal marrow I and VI run exclusively in the intercostal space (ICS) reaching the sternum. ICN VII to X cross in the costal arch and the fibrous layer between the abdominal transverse muscles and the internal oblique muscles. ICN IX and XII come from the open intercostal space to each of the muscles mentioned above.

The ICN supply the autonomic thoracic and abdominal muscles and the skin of the thorax and abdomen to the inguinal ligament and to the region of the hip, mural pleura, the mural peritoneum of the lateral and anterior wall.

Odontogenic irritations on intercostal nerves may cause irritations of the spinal marrow:

1. The 8th odonton on TH-1 and TH-2 (upper intercostal nerves), the upper odontons 4, 5 and the lower odontons 6, 7 on TH-3 and TH-4 (upper intercostal nerves).
2. The 8th odonton on TH-5, TH-6, TH-7 (middle intercostal nerves), the 3rd odonton on TH-8, TH-9, and TH-10 (lower intercostal nerves), the upper odontons 6, 7 and the lower odontons 4, 5 on TH-11, TH-12 (lowest intercostal nerves).
3. The intercostal nerves innervate muscular, cutaneous, pleural and peritoneal branches of the body.

Odontogenic Irritations to the Cerebrum

Irritations from the odontons to the cerebrum can affect 3 measurement values:

1. Thalamus opticus GB-4 in the diencephalon which involves the function of speech and the sleep centers GB-16 for deep sleep.
2. Formatio reticularis in the mesencephalon GB-17 is the center of activity where the center of consciousness is situated and the sleep and wake center GB-11. All fibers of sensual performances such as palpation, pain, temperature, hearing and seeing emit branches to the formatio reticularis. The formatio reticularis is responsible for the coordination of all autonomic functions of the skeletal muscles and for the regulation of the tone of the muscles. It also regulates tone; the retarding component is responsible for the induction of sleep while the activating system regulates the degree of consciousness.

   The center for sleep and wake rhythm GB-11 in the mesencephalon helps recharge the battery of our body. The depth of sleep is governed by the sleep center in the thalamus and by the formatio reticularis, while regular sleep and wake rhythm is governed by a special center in the mesencephalon.
3. Medulla oblongata UB-10 is the center for cardiac activity for blood pressure, coughing, vomiting and for inspiration and expiration. The pons UB-9 in the center is for panting respiration.

Odontogenic Irritations on the Joints

One irritated odonton can functionally disturb only one joint or a portion of a joint where the pain will then be felt. The odontogenic articular irritation can be characterized by a pain of a joint, but it can be irritated even without pain so that only the x-ray will show it.

Odontogenic Irritations on the Reflexes

Organic nerve diseases affect several reflexes which will change pathologically whereas in odontogenic focus-related dysreflexia affects mostly one or a few reflexes are changed with pathologic changes being only slight.

The 8th Odonton as Related to Other Disturbances

The upper wisdom tooth has, according to Voll, an effect on the cerebrum, especially after puberty. Irregular behavior such as fits of rage, negative influence of psychic life on the thymopsyche, accompanied by bad moods, disgruntleness, inactivity, lack of stimulation, even depression, disturbances of emotional and mental life or with introvertedness and lack of social contact are caused by irritation of the limbic system.

The 8th odonton is related to the ears and the heart: the right 8th odonton to the right ear and the right part of the heart, the left to the left ear and the left part of the heart. The upper wisdom teeth are related to the small intestine. In the course of enzyme formation and fermentation in the small intestine, large quantities of energy are produced for the maintenance of the body's energy balance. The lower wisdom teeth are related to the large intestine and may be the cause of chronic constipation.

A unilateral occurrence of blisters are associated with focal disturbances of the 8th odonton or an impacted wisdom tooth. In contrast, general blisters on the tongue may be due to intestinal disturbances related to a metabolic malfunction.

DENTAL THERAPY

Holistic Dental Therapy

Dental therapy plays an important role in EAV. Dental foci of infection in most instances can cause other functions of the body to be affected. These are discussed in the first part of the chapter. The dentist must avail himself of more knowledge than is taught in a dental school. He must be holistically orientated, responsible for diagnosing, treating and practicing preventive dentistry. Preventive dentistry to him is preventing a foci of infection from spreading from the teeth to the rest of the body's tissues or vice versa. Knowledge of anatomy, physiology, neurology, bacteriology, pharmacology, etc., which he has seldom used in practice, must be reviewed thoroughly and now put to good use.

Understanding the relationship of the tonsils, sinuses, joints, vertebrae, muscles, nerves, etc., must be understood in order to be a holistic dentist. Postural analysis and other disciplines such as kinesiology, cranial osteopathy, Oriental medicine, ultrasound therapy and biomagnets are like EAV, a total composite of healing.

It is again imperative that those who want to learn more about acupuncture take a formal course from Voll and Khoe. It is not my intention to teach you about electro-acupuncture but merely to acquaint you with the importance it has as a discipline in the healing arts in dentistry. In order for you to learn and understand, you must study and practice this seven days a week.

Measurement Points in EAV for Individual Jaw Sections

The dentist must acquaint himself with the basic measurement points and EAV application to diseases and dysfunctions. Lymph measurement point 2 is located caudally on the volar surface of the second joint of each thumb. When there is an indicator drop measurement on this point, that side has a dental irritation.

Anterior upper jaw, 1st to 4th odontons, left and right side equals GV-25.

Anterior lower jaw, 1st to 4th odontons, left and right equals CV-24.

Right lateral upper jaw, 5th to 8th odontons equals St-7 right.

Left lateral upper jaw, 5th to 8th odontons equals St-7 left.

Left lateral lower jaw, 5th to 8th odontons equals St-8 left.

Right lateral lower jaw, 5th to 8th odontons equals St-8 right.

Dental Foci of Infection

The relation between a pair of organs, paranasal sinuses, tonsils and others is not one way. The organs in the body may irritate the organs of the head and vice versa. For example, a focated wisdom tooth or a residual ostitis in a toothless wisdom odonton area or a scar tissue may interfere with an otherwise excellent heart therapy because the focal toxins of the 8th odonton may react with the heart. Another example: a chronic inflammation of the lower odontons 1 and 2 may cause constant rectal, anal canal and urinary bladder infections which may make other treatments fail because the doctor is unaware of the connection.

These dental foci of infections may include:

1. Scars in the gingivae to the fields of disturbances . . . A scar tissue due to a surgical contraction of the floor of the mouth . . . A scar due to an operation of the jaw sinus after a Caldwell Luc and after Denker. When measuring a jaw section with a reading of 82 to 88 plus indicator drop and the tooth found to be normal

upon normal conventional dental testings, a field of disturbances from a scar on the gingivae should be tested. Stroke the scar with the stylus electrode and compare it with the reading of the surrounding areas. At the point of the highest value, inject impletol and then test lymph measurement point 2 and the remote organ irritation. Lymph 2 and the irritated organ should show lower measurement values, indicating that the foci of infection was from the scar itself. Some people who are allergic to caffeine should take hyaluronidase, thiosinamine, graphites or hepar sulfuricum. The tolerance of impletol may be tested on the arteries MPcirculation- 9.

2. Dental restorations such as:
   a. Acrylic, autoacrylic, polyvinyl acrylic
   b. Gold
   c. Amalgam, copper amalgam
   d. Chrome — cobalt metal in partial prosthesis
   e. Paladium — gold in porcelain fused to metal restorations
   f. Resin materials filling
   g. Silicate filling

3. Dental cements:
   a. Zinc oxide cement
   b. Phosphoric acid cement
   c. Carboxylate cement
   d. Root canal cements

4. Dental Disease:
   a. Gingivitis
   b. Caries
   c. Ostitis
   d. Pulpitis

Testing a Dental Foci of Infection with Homeopathic Remedies

When testing lymph 2 with one having an ID, you have located a DENTAL FOCI OF INFECTION. Match the remedy on the DERMATRON until the DIAGNOSTIC OHMMETER registers 50. This will indicate what homeopathic remedy is good for this malady. If a nosode is used, this will indicate the type of infection that the patient has. Homeopathic remedies should be tested. Nosodes can be used and combined with other remedies to produce the best results. If values register over 82, then low dilution from D3 and up are used for acute inflammation. Determine the dosage by measuring the selected remedy or nosodes on lymph 2 until the normal value of 50 is attained. This is the correct dosage for this patient.

Intramuscular injections are more effective than globule of the same dilutions. Inject and follow this with 5 globules per hour until the pain has subsided. Then administer 5 globules every 3 hours for the next day and then 4 globules four times a day for one week.

The patient is seen within a week for a reassessment of the dosages. It is best that the patient is seen twice on the first day for an injection of the remedies, approximately 8 hours apart.

When the lymph measurement point 2 and its associated remote organs return to 50 and stay there, then there is no need for further treatments. If upon testing more than 3 ampules of a teeth nosode like "ostitis" or "pulpitis" in D-3 are necessary to bring the point to 50, an extraction is usually indicated. In these cases, you can expect a longer time lapse in treatment.

Injections intramuscularly should be given once to twice a week for the first week followed by globules of 6 once or twice a week the following weeks. Patients should have their dosages changed once a week.

Homeopathic remedies and nosodes should be sucked and not swallowed with liquid.

TMJ Dental Irritation

A dental related irritation is that of the temporomandibular joint. When the joint articulation measurement point 3 registers an INDICATOR DROP, then the temporomandibular joint or the first and second cervical vertebrae may be affected. If further testing of measurement point 23 on the triple warmer meridian of the upper compartment of the TMJ and the measurement point on stomach 2 in the lower capsule show a difference of 10 reading from one side to the other, the side of the greatest deviation indicates a premature occlusion or TMJ involvement. The usual reading is 84-85 without an indicator drop. Medication and irritated cranial nerves must be investigated. The trigeminal V Gbl-3, vestibulocochlear VIII SI-18, glosso-pharyngeal IX TW-22 and the hypoglossal XII nerves St-5a may be involved. Neuralgias of vari-ous cranial nerves — painful sensations in the naso-pharyngeal space, acoustic disturbances, dizziness, occasional tubal stenosis, parasthesia

NOTES

and even pains of the tongue as well as the lack of changes of sensitivity of taste and the disturbances of mastication of the jaw-movement may be experienced.

First the occlusion, usually the mandibular molars, must be checked for a prematurity on the side of the greatest difference of values. Again measure triple warmer 23 and stomach 2 after the prematurity is removed. Jankelson's myomonitor can be used to spot the prematurity. If the values of both joint measurements are equal, the problem is removed. Also check joint degeneration measurement point 3 and compare it to the original readings. If the values are less than the originals without an indicator drop, the condition is improving. If the compared reading shows little improvement, then homeopathic remedies or nosodes must be used.

By reducing the irritated nerve measurement values to 50 the irritated symptoms can be reduced. However, this may offer only temporary relief from pain without the use of medication.

Ultrasound therapy, as an alternative method, can be used on the acupuncture measurement points of the trigeminal V, vestibulocochlear VIII, glossopharyngeal IX and hypoglossal nerve XII. Use V2 watt with a Vultrasound head on these nerve acupuncture points.

Trigeminal Neuralgia — (Tic Douleroux)

Nerve disorders involving the fifth cranial nerve and formerly known as Tic Douleroux have plagued neurologists, otolaryngologists, dentists and even psychiatrists. Cortisone, alcohol and procaine injections, surgery and occlusal splinting have been used with varying success. The following is a brief summary of the procedure of diagnosing and treating trigeminal neuralgia:

Diagnosis

Check allergy measurement point 3. This mea-surement point is on the 3rd knuckle on the middle finger on the ulnar side. The allergy point 3 represents allergic irritations of the skin of the head or the mucosa, organs of the head, oral cavity, nasal and paranasal sinus (drippy nose) and allergic irritations from dental materials. If there is an indicator drop, one or several of the above are involved. The next measurement point is the nerve degeneration MP-3a — the autonomic parasympathetic ganglia (cranial division of the autonomic system). The parasympathetic nervous system is used to build up and keep in reverse energy the body needs while the sympathetic nerve uses the energy throughout the day.

If this cranial ganglia shows an indicator drop, the following ganglia should be checked:

1. The pterygopalatine ganglion is the most important of the four. It can be irritated by chronic inflammation of the ethmoidal sinuses (with ID on lymph 3). Some of the symptoms can be from an increased flow of tears from the eye on the side of the sinus focus, lateral mucus secretion of the nose, the gums and the maxillary sinus St-5 and cavernous sinus may also irritate the pterygopalatine ganglion.
2. The ciliary ganglion disturbances can result in a unilateral narrowing of the pupil (a ocaria). The oculomotor, trigeminal nerve GB-MP-3 and the cavernous sinus can influence celiac ganglion disturbances.
3. The oticum ganglion, SI-MP-18a, increases the salivation and abnormal sensation of taste. The glossopharyngeal nerve and the trigeminal nerve are affected.
4. The submandibular ganglion, St-MP-83, controls an increase or a decrease in salivation which is dependent on the level of stress.

The control measurement point of the cranial nerves should be tested. This is situated on nerve degeneration MP-4. If this shows an indicator drop, the individual cranial nerves should be checked. The trigeminal and facial nerves should be measured. The wisdom tooth should also be evaluated.

Treatment (according to Voll)

1. Check for viruses of the nervous system like herpes virus, tularaemia, and smallpox (variola), chicken pox, toxoplasmose.
2. Check for poisons irritating the nervous system like silver amalgam, chrom-cobalt-molybdenum, venyl polymerisat, acaryophyllum, and other chemical substances used in dentistry. Check for insecticides.
3. Give homeopathic organ preparation, nervus trigeminus (for the 5th nerve) subcutaneously, or magnesium fluoratum, calcium, potassium, and sodium fluoride.
4. Use a small roller 1 or 2 HZ, 2 intensity and reduce the energy from here. With the small roller, have the patient roll up and down from

the ear out until the pain is relieved. When rolling near the corner of the eye, have the patient observe if there is flickering — if so, your HZ is too high and should be reduced.

Treatment (according to Khoe)

1. On the left side of the face, try either magnesium fluoratum, calcium potassium or sodium fluoride.
2. Inject mezereum in St-MP-5; LI-MP-18.
3. Kyolic (garlic) and dong quai, 4 capsules 4 times a day; ume (extract or pellets), 4 pellets 4 times a day; arnica lotion or EE oils used as a conducting media with the ultrasound^— large head and low voltage (according to Kho'e).
4. Give vitamin E, selenium and vitamin C granules, 10 grams.
5. No smoking and drinking are allowed.

It is not necessary to give all of the above. Select the remedy or nosode which gives the best reading on Voll's instrument.

Therapy (according to Khoe)

1. Inject Pons BL-MP-9 with vitamin B-12 on both sides. If this doesn't work, inject V2 cc of vitamin B-12 on the trigger points of the LI-MP-10 and LI-MP-17a at the angle of the jaw. You can use a roller at 2 HZ frequency or ultrasound (according to Voll).
2. Also inject vitamin B-12 on GBL-MP-3, superior to the upper compartment of the TMJ over the zygomatic bone.
3. Also place needles on the ophthalmic division of V nerve measurement point, GBL-MP-34 and St-MP-36 (on the leg).
4. Ultrasound for 3 minutes each the autonomic division, LI-MP-15, BL-MP-2, LI-MP-20 and the second division St-MP-3, SI-MP-18, CVMP- 24 and TW-MP-18.
5. Then give vitamin C, I.V., 12 grams in 100 cc with 5% glucose in water, once a day.

When practicing a therapy according to Khoe that proves successful, stop this therapy. You need not continue the steps of the therapy. It is important that the doctor not overtreat the patient. When the patient receives immediate relief, stick to that therapy. If not, continue to take other steps. It will take 8 to 10 weeks to achieve lasting results.

According to Voll, you have to continue the treatment systematically for 10 weeks. The pain may be gone after the first injections, but you need to continue treatments so the body can bring out all the poisons and viruses in the nerve or in other parts of the body. If you give up soon after the pain has gone, it may return.

Tooth Testing (according to Voll)

When an indicator drop is measured on dental point lymph MP-2 or its particular jaw section, the individual tooth of that jaw section must be tested as a focus of irritation. The following procedures can be followed on the Dermatron:
Sedate to 50 Lymph MP-2:

1. Depress top row first button, energy.
2. Press in waveswing.
3. Adjust to intensity 3.
4. Set frequency to HZ-7.
5. Press the button of the red stylus electrode 2 times and press down on the junction of the gum and tooth root being tested.
6. Then measure again lymph 2.
7. If the indicator rises past 50 on lymph MP-2, the irritation to the organ or tissue system is caused by the focated tooth.

Teeth Irritation

When testing the terminal measuring points on the hands and all points show an indicator drop, an odontogenic focus of infection is indicated. The teeth can also be irritated by bacterial infections such as streptococcus and staphylococcus.

Teeth irritation can cause:

1. Frontal sinus can control teeth 1, 2, 3; centrals, laterals. Teeth 6, 7 can cause problems on the left breast.
2. Headaches can be caused by infections from any of the teeth.
3. Teeth 1 of the uppers and lowers can cause urinary bladder problems. Clinically observe if there are gum infections, capping, root canals and bridges on the lower and upper anterior teeth. Use ultrasound (by Khoe) with the large head. Check the bladder and kidney and for cancer in the prostate. Neutralize these points with nosodes.
4. Asthma can be caused by irritations of the upper 4, 5 (1st and 2nd bicuspids), lower 6, 7 (1st and 2nd molars). Check the measurement point, LI-MP-20, ethmoid point for all cases of asthma.
5. The anterior part of the eye can be influenced from the lower cuspid and the retina from the

upper cuspid. If the eye is going blind, stimulate the MP eye, Ly-MP-2a. If there is a high reading on the liver, allergy point and gallbladder, then check the cuspids on both sides with nosodes. Also test for inflammation on the optic nerve II from a focus of infection from the upper 3rd odonton.

6. If the patient has postoperative bleeding from extraction or residual ostitis, give magnesium muriaticum D-4 and calcium carbonicum D-6, 3 globules twice a day after meals for several days. If the globules are given 2-3 days before the extraction you can *avoid* bleeding.

Tooth Therapy (according to Khoe)

It is the responsibility of the dentist to practice preventive therapy as well as crisis treatment. When testing the teeth for a focus infection and the readings register 90 plus when the probe is placed on the roots, treat the tooth with ultrasound for 10 minutes once a week. If the tooth is bad, treat twice a week. Use the large ultrasound head on the face over the treated teeth. Treat even if the tooth is not sensitive to percussion and is negative on the x-rays. Measure these values once a week to see if these measurements are reduced to 50 or in the range from 50-65 without an indicator drop.

Toothaches (according to Khoe)

There are several alternatives to relieving a toothache besides the normal dental technique.

1. Inject B-12 in the toothache point in the ear-lobes.
2. Inject B-12 in LI-MP-4 — the master toothache point.
3. Inject B-12 in allergy MP-3.
4. Inject B-12 in stomach MP-3, glandular submandibulars diagonally distal to stomach MP-8 on the inferior border of the mandible.
5. If the patient is unable to be treated in the office, have him place a clothes pin between the earlobe and its attachment to the face for ten minutes.

Sensitive Teeth (according to Voll)

If upon testing MP-Ly-2 (or the jaw section) and the tooth is inflamed, sedate MP-Ly-2 and acupuncture measure jaw section to 50 for pain relief and match the appropriate nosodes for this on Ly-2 and/or the local MP for the odonton.

Match chronic or acute pulpitis nosode preparation, kieferostitis (ostitis) or gangranose pulpa (granulomous pulp) for a tooth that is sensitive to percussion. Also zahnfleischtasche (pockets in gums) and zahnwurzelgranulom (granulation tissue around roots) should be considered. Other nosodes are gingivitis, gingivitis ulceros, gingivitis necrotic, stomatitis, paradontose, paradontose with diabetes. Follow this with a miniroller attached to the red positive plug with the patient holding the negative brass electrode. The frequency is set from 8 HZ and the intensity set at 1. The second sedation button is depressed. Roll the gingivae over the roots of the tooth for ten minutes over the labial and lingual surfaces.

Postoperative Extractions, Hematomas, Swelling and Pain (according to Voll)

It is useful to reduce stasis in the lymphatic vessels and glands especially after extractions. In cases of hematomas and swelling, the following procedures using oscillating low-frequency therapy have proved to be effective:

1. Depress energy button 1 (waveswing).
2. Set frequency to 8 HZ.
3. Adjust intensity to the patient's tolerance.
4. Use a large roller with red cord in positive (black plug is negative).
5. Roll the side of the cheek and the neck where the extraction was done and Ly-MP-2, 11, 12, 13, 14.
6. Sedate with button 2.
7. Set frequency to 3.8 HZ.
8. Set intensity at 2 (or less, especially when the eyes are flickering).

Fevers (according to Voll)

When a patient is experiencing a high temperature, you can try to reduce the high values measured hand to hand with the Dermatron with a reading of 95-93 down to 88. Use the 2nd button, the positive spike and lower the intensity (1-3) as always, in sedation therapy. You cannot bring the measurement down to 50. You can bring them down to maybe 88 and then they will increase again. When it begins to increase, stop the Dermatron treatment immediately. According to Khoe, you can inject B-12 or use ultrasound on LI-MP-11 bilaterally and GV-MP-14.

Drippy Nose (according to Khoe)

The dentist must often work on a patient whose oral cavity has a drippy nose syndrome. By reducing these measurement points to 50 on Ly-MP-13, GV-14, 15, 20, and allergy 3, the dentist can control most postnasal drip and reduce fevers within 15 minutes.

1. Depress 2nd button, sedation.
2. Set frequency to 3.8 HZ.
3. Set intensity to 1.
4. Use ultrasound or inject B-12 according to Khoe into these measurement points as an alternative.

Sore Throat (according to Khoe)

Sore throats can be controlled by sedation therapy on measurement points CV-22, 23, deep cervical lymph nodes TW-16a, CV-17 between the nipples, LI-11 on the arm below the elbow and rolling Lu-1-9. If the sore throat is not relieved, inject B-12 subcutaneously on stomach-plexus 8c.

Earaches (according to Voll)

Ear problem can be caused by illness of the middle ear TW-17 and the internal ear TW-18. In treating ear problems, the following should be evaluated:

1. Small childhood infections, staphylococcus.
2. Homeopathic mercurusol 6X, 4 globules TID before meals helps.
3. Sedate small intestine control point to 50 on the same side of earache and TW-17 and 18, the MP's of the middle and inner ears.
4. The deep cervical lymph nodes can be sedated with the roller on TW-16a.

The ear is related to the wisdom teeth and can affect the heart, duodenum and other parts of the small intestine. Earaches are related to the meninges TW-19 and the ear MP-Ly-1-1.

For those patients who have tinnitus or who are hard of hearing, check these points of measurement and the ductuli bilifori:

1. Sphenoid sinus.
2. Ductuli bilifori of the liver lobe on the foot, GBL-MP-41.
3. Ki-3 (Chinese point) posterior to the medial maleolus of the ankle of the foot.
4. Small intestine MP-2, 3 on the hand.
5. Ear M P - L y - 1 - 1.
6. Labyrinth — TW-MP-17a behind the ear.
7. Cochlea — back of the ear.
8. Middle ear — TW-MP-17.
9. Mastoid cells —TW-16a.
10. With the roller, use sedation therapy if there is inflammation, and use tonification if there is degeneration. An alternative is to use ultrasound with high wattage stroking behind the ear and around it (according to Khoe).

NOTES

CONCLUSION

Electro-acupuncture by Voll has made its presence known in preventive medicine and dentistry today. Until recently, it was difficult to treat the patient who showed definite symptoms because there was a problem in determining the status of the dysfunction and disease in the patient. There was no way to accurately measure the correct dose, the effectiveness of the medication used or whether one was dealing with irritation, inflammation or degeneration.

The use of laboratory tests and x-rays has revealed certain illness present in a crisis stage of development. With EAV, one is able to measure the progress of the treatment of not only electroacupuncture therapy but that of other disciplines. It has enabled the dentist to expand his responsibility in treating the whole health as related to the odontons. It further makes the dentist recognize that he may be introducing irritating materials in the oral cavity which may create serious health problems in the future. Dentists can now use all the science he has learned in school and put it to practical use.

New avenues of treatment are opened without using addicting drugs in helping his patients holistically. In order to continue his personal growth in holistic health, the dentist must expand his horizons in research, studying and practicing seven days a week. He must become familiar with all disciplines of natural health in order to fulfill the mental, spiritual and physical aspects of the healing profession. If he is willing to do this, he will become the total health orientated dentist and realize his true potential in his profession.

BIBLIOGRAPHY

Khoe, Willem H,, M.D., "Referred Pain: A Holistic Approach in Acupuncture." *American Journal of Acupuncture.* Vol. 6, No. 1. March 1978.

Leonhardt, H,, M.D., translated by Helga Sarkisyauz, An *Introduction to Electro-Acupuncture According to Voll.* 1976.

Voll, Reinhold, M.D., *Topographic Positions of the Measurement Points in Electro-Acupuncture.* Illus. Vol. I. 1976.

Voll, Reinhold, M.D., *Topographic Positions at the Measurement Points in Electro-Acupuncture.* Textual Vol. I. 1977.

Voll, Reinhold, M.D., *Topographic Positions of the Measurement Points in Electro-Acupuncture.* Illus. Vol. II. 1977.

Voll, Reinhold, M.D., *Textual and Illustrated.* Vol. III. 1978.

Voll, Reinhold, M.D., *1st Supplement to the Four Volumes on the Topographic Positions of the Measurement Points in Electro-Acupuncture (EAV).* 1978.

Voll, Reinhold, M.D., *Interrelations of Odontons and Tonsils to Organs, Field of Disturbances and Tissue Systems.* Reading copy. 1978.

Voll, Reinhold, M.D., "Electro-Acupuncture According to Voll." *American Journal of Acupuncture, Special Issue.* 1978.

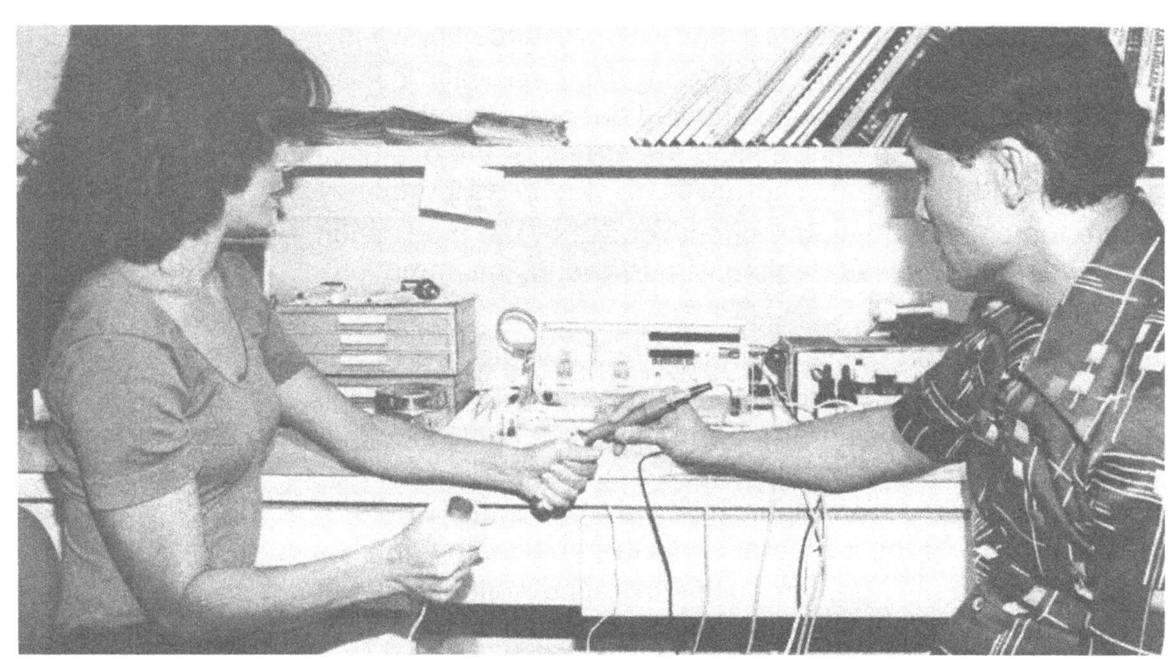

Patient's energy should record 82 on diagnostic meter before acupuncture points are measured.

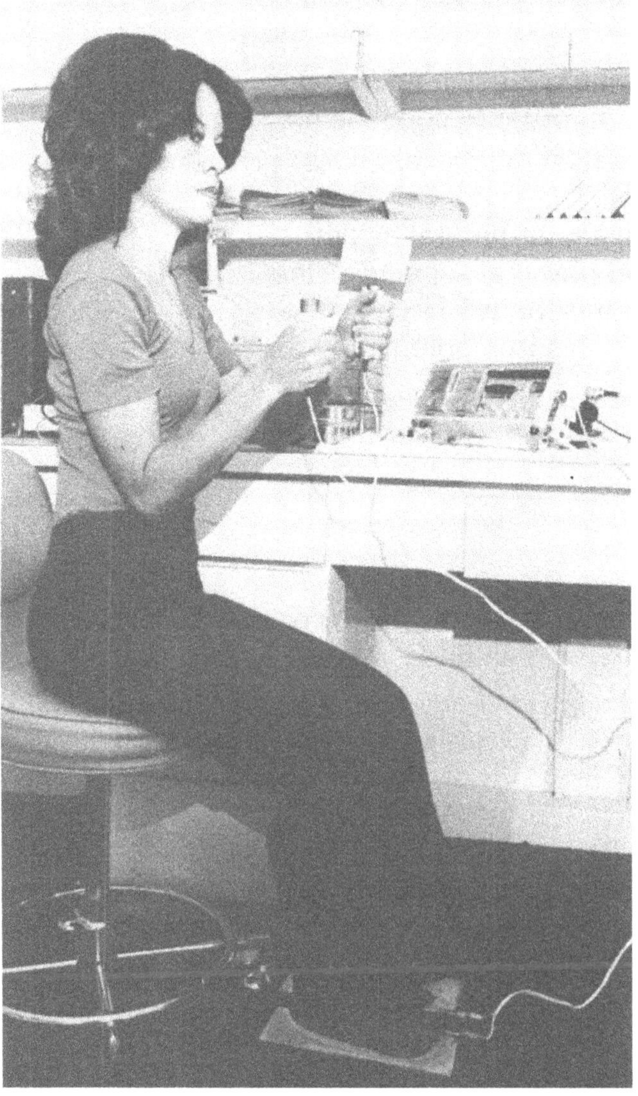

Four quadrants of the body are measured and energized or sedated.

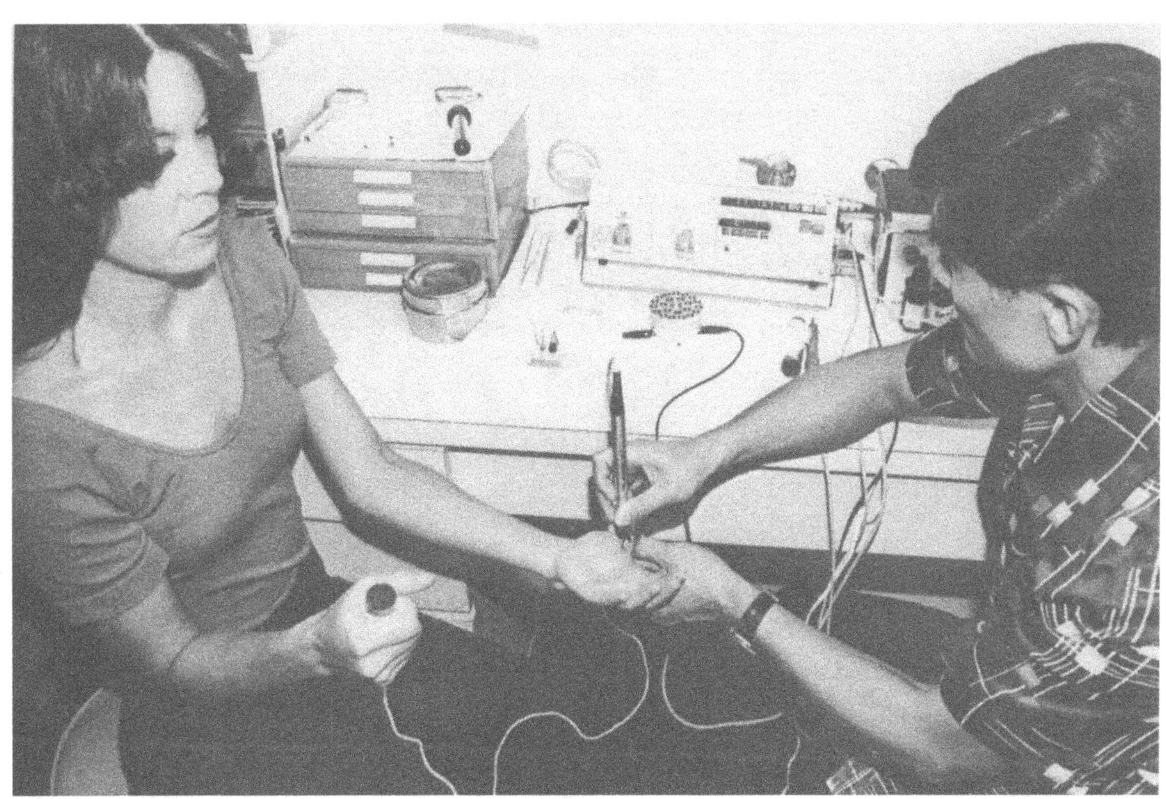

Dental Lymph MP-2 is measured.

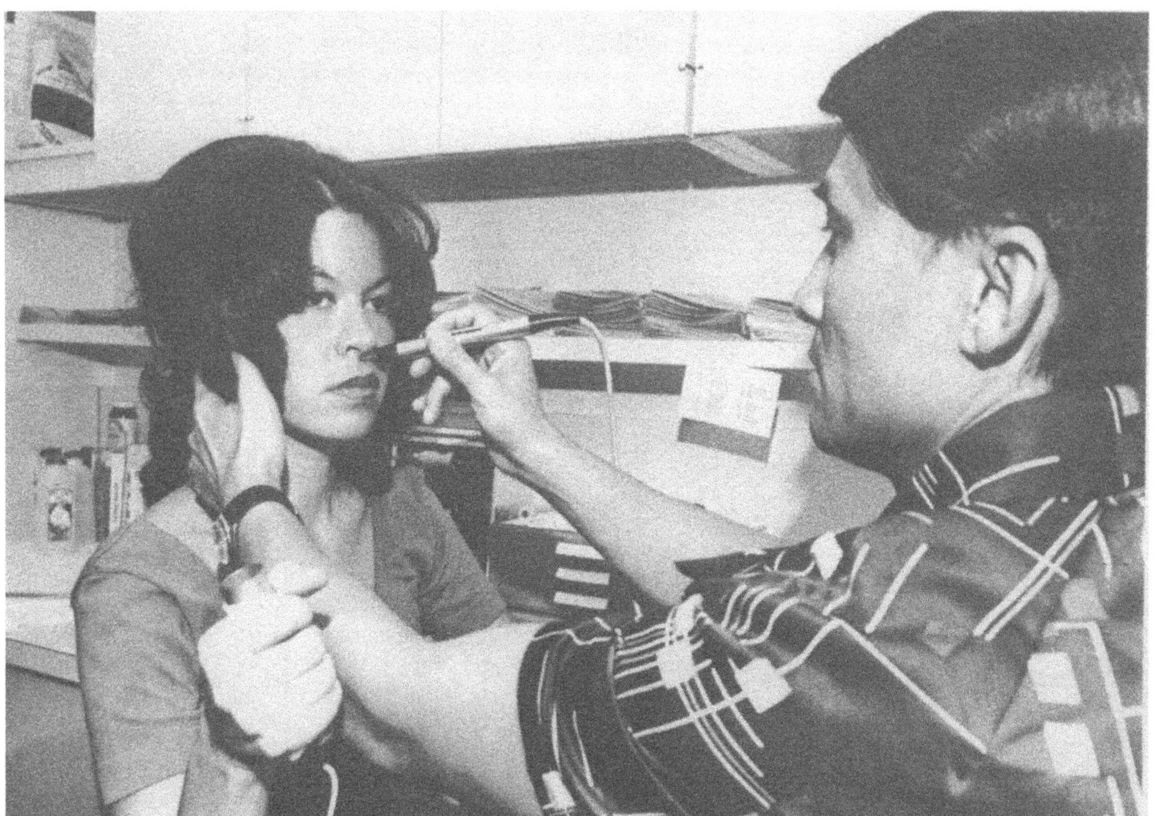

Governing MP-25 is measured for energetic imbalance of upper 1st bicuspid to 1st bicuspid

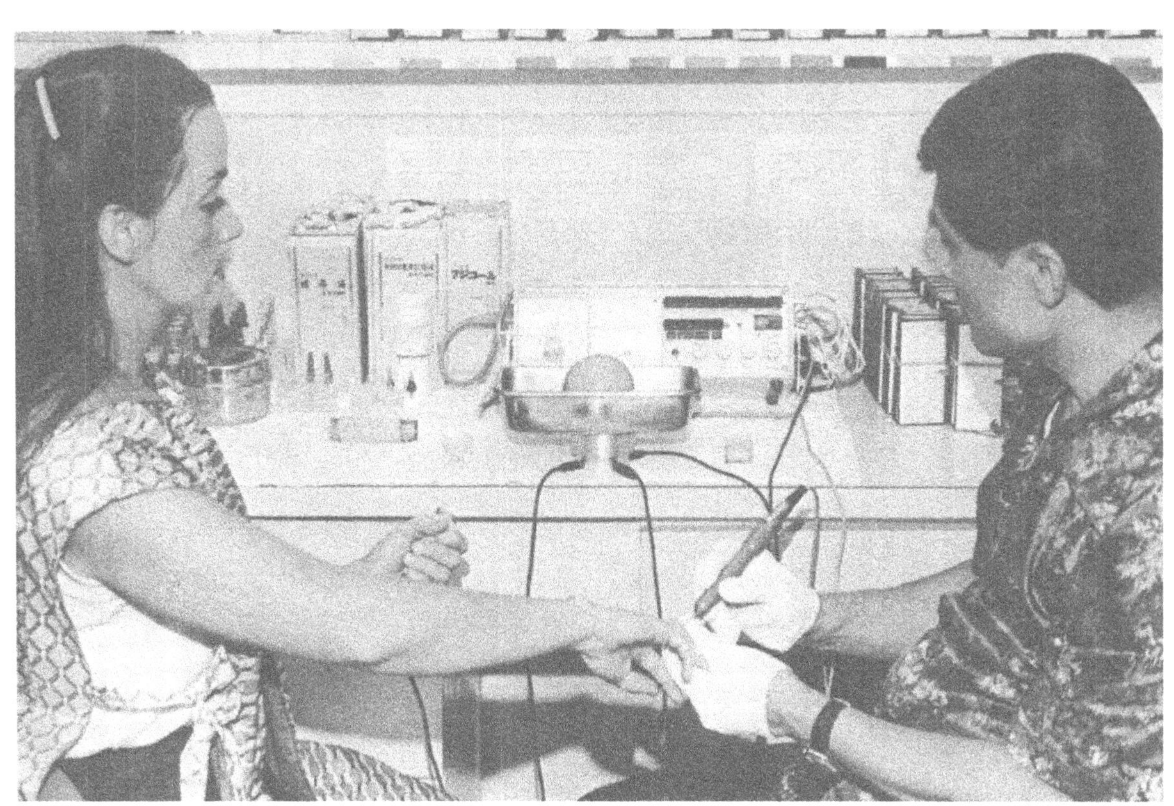

Orange fruit measured on allergy control measurement point.

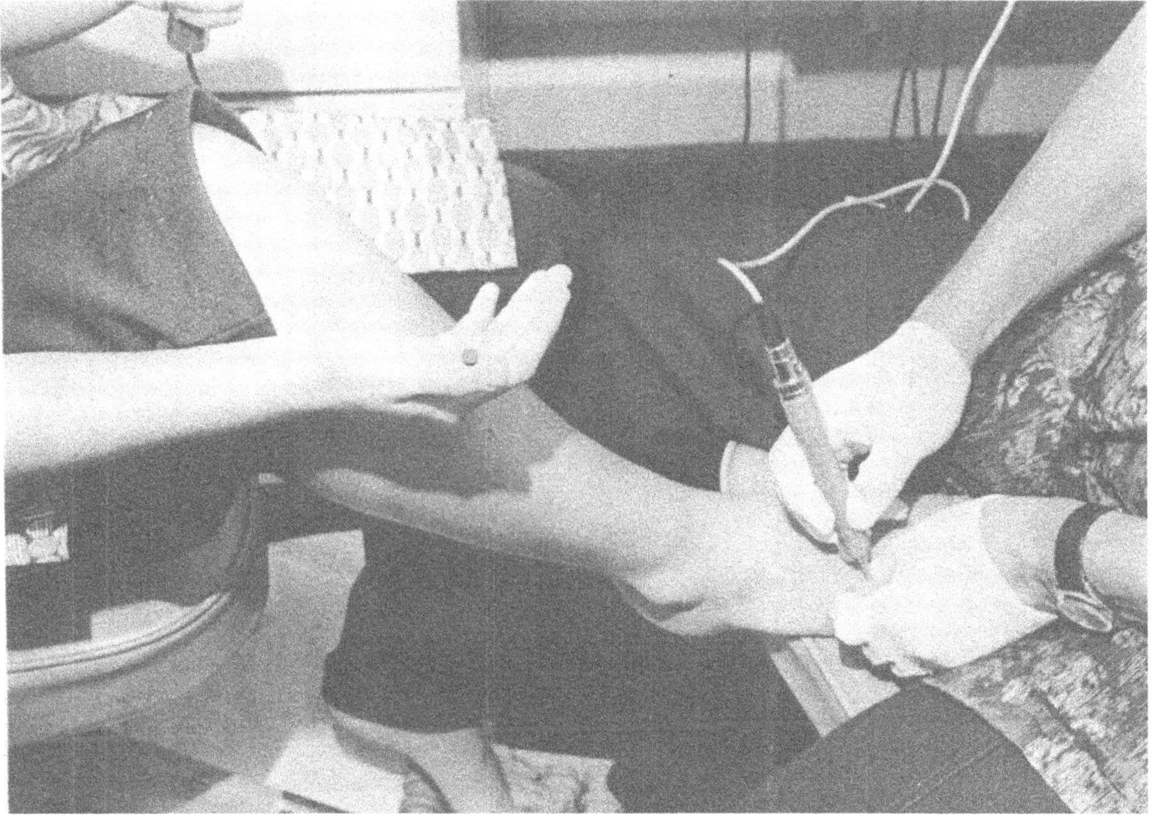

Magnet analyzer placed on tooth and lymph MP-2 measured.

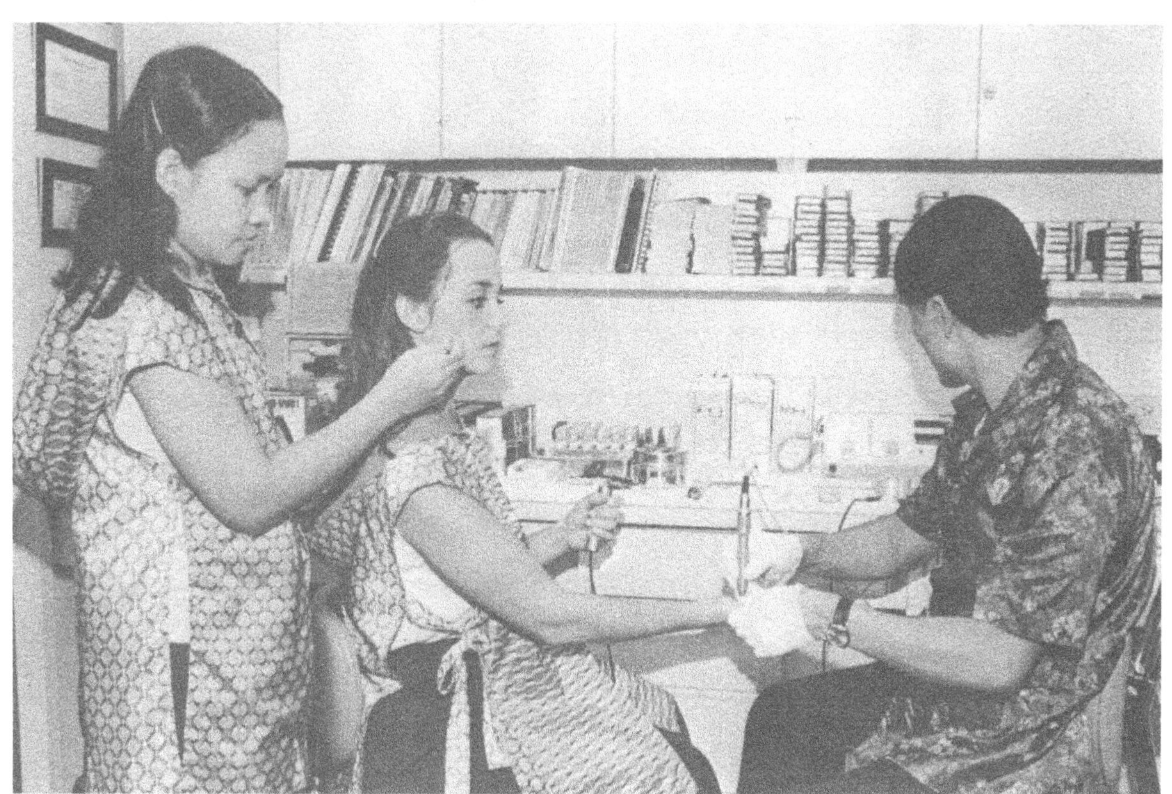

Lymph MP-1-1 ear with magnet and kidney CMP on the foot measured with dermatron. If meter reads 50, the ear is the cause of the irritation to the kidney.

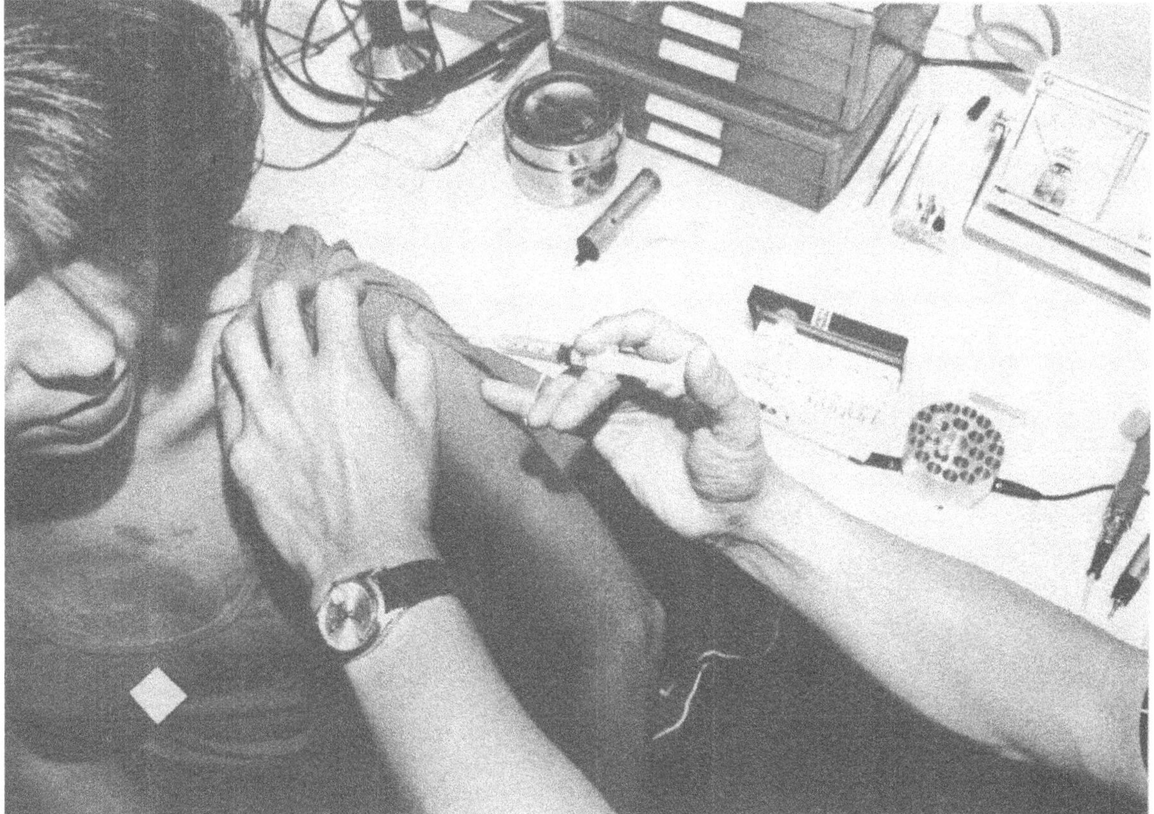

Homeopathic remedies injected intramuscularly.

NOTES

John K. Char, D.D.S., the founder of Nutri-Kinetic Dynamics, Inc., has been deeply involved in the future of preventive dentistry. His books, **Holistic Dentistry Volumes** I and II and **Electro-Acupuncture for Dentistry**, illustrate the practical use of combining the ancient sciences with modern technology in treating dental stresses and the TMJ syndrome as it relates to the total body.

Dr. Char graduated from the Creighton School of Dentistry and has been practicing preventive dentistry for 19 years. His practice was first publicized in the cover story of the April 1978 issue of **Dental Survey.** Dr. Char has studied and researched the holistic sciences in Germany under Dr. Reinhold Voll, as well as under Viola Frymann, D.O. and Willem Khoe, M.D. Over 2000 hours of post-graduate studies and research have gone into producing the volume on Holistic Dentistry. Dr. Char has lectured to health organizations, dental study groups, hospitals, dental societies and dental state conventions. He also has been on KNDI and K-108 radio shows, KHON and KHET television programs and interviewed in the Hawaii Health and the Honolulu Star-Bulletin newspapers. Dr. Char has served on the teaching staff at St. Francis Hospital, Queen's Hospital, and Kapiolani Dental Assistant School. His local dental accomplishments have been to serve as founder and president of the Leeward Prosthetics Study Group, president of the Western Study Group of Combined Therapy, president of the American Endodontic Society of Hawaii, president of the Holistic Dental Study Group, and president of the Honolulu County Dental Society. He has served as a chairman for the committee to provide dental relief for the orphanage children in Korea, the Honolulu County Ethics Committee, the Honolulu County Expanded Duties Auxiliary Personnel, the Honolulu County Executive Committee, the Academy of Mandibular Kinesiology, and the Honolulu County Dental Society. He has also served as an advisor to the University of Hawaii School of Hygiene.

Dr. Char has organized annual seminars in Hawaii — Mandibular Kinesiology and steopathy in the Cranial Field for dentists. He now serves on the Board of Directors for the American Endodontic Society and is a charter member of the Holistic Dental Association International. He is a member of the American Dental Association, Academy of General Dentistry, Western Study Group of Combined Therapy, National Health Federation, Cranial Academy Associate, Acupuncture Research Institute, International Association of Electro-Acupuncture — Hawaii, American Endodontic Society, and the Holistic Dental Association International.

His civil awards include Outstanding Men of American awards 1969, 1971, Who's Who in the West 1970-1971 and Congress Director for the XXVI Junior Chamber International World Congress in 1967. He has won every major award as an officer and member in the United States Jaycees as well as an international involvement award in 1970. As President of the Honolulu Chinese Jaycees, Dr. Char received the Dillingham award and Giessenbier memorial trophy for the most outstanding president and chapter in the State of Hawaii in 1968. In 1967, he joined the exclusive United States Jaycees President's Club and the Junior Chamber International Senate in 1971.

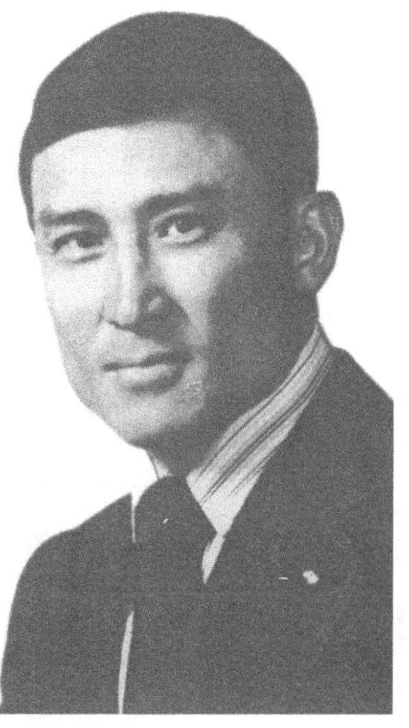

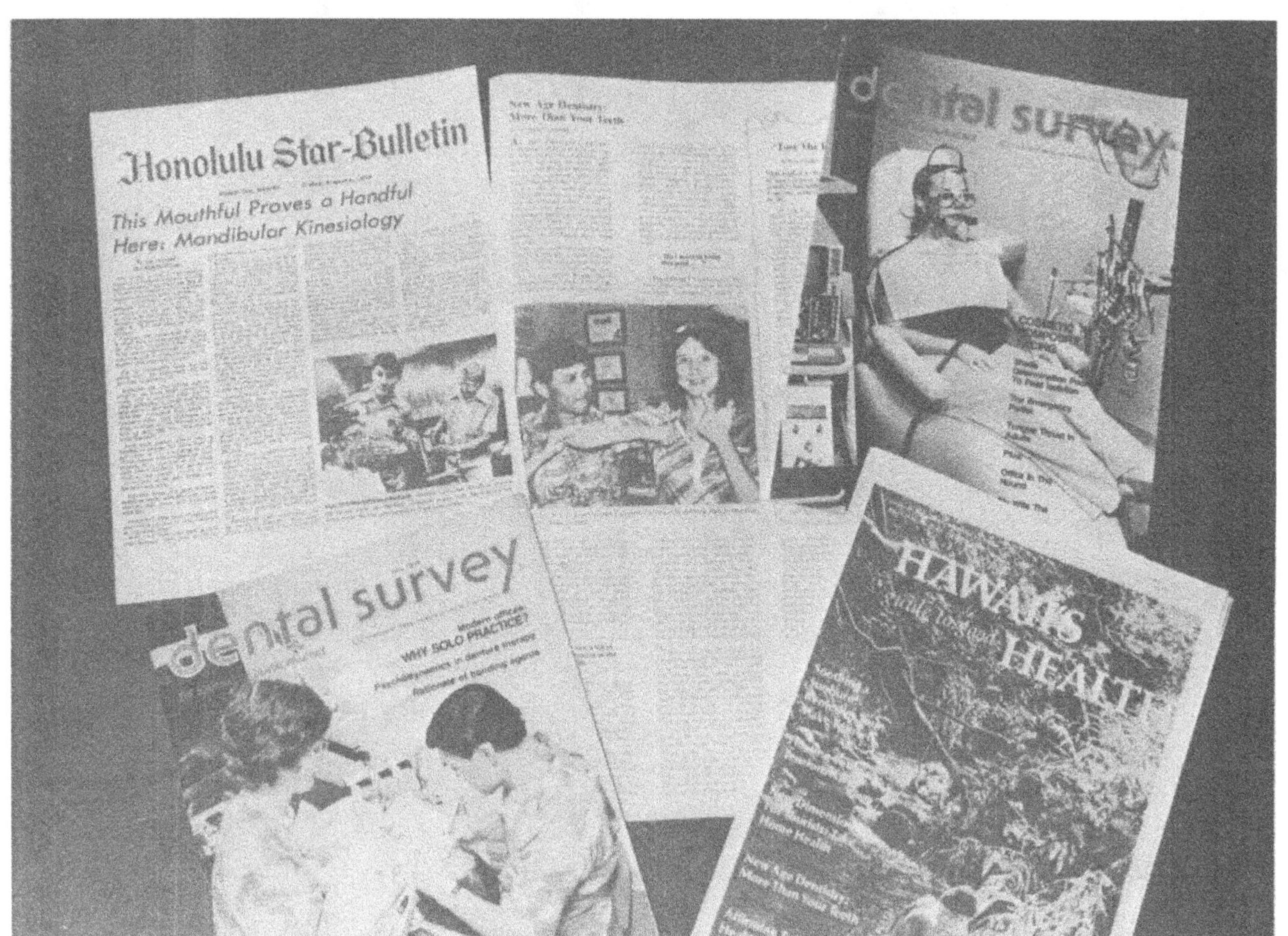
Honolulu Star-Bulletin
This Mouthful Proves a Handful Here: Mandibular Kinesiology
dental survey
dental survey
WHY SOLO PRACTICE?
HAWAII'S HEALTH

www.ingramcontent.com/pod-product-compliance
Lightning Source LLC
Chambersburg PA
CBHW081542220326
41598CB00036B/6531

* 9 7 8 1 9 3 8 0 3 4 0 2 2 *